The Pilates Body

The Ultimate At-Home Guide to Strengthening, Lengthening,
and Toning Your Body—Without Machines

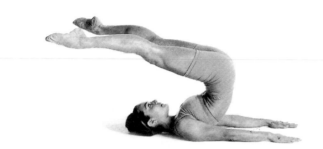

The
Pilates
Body

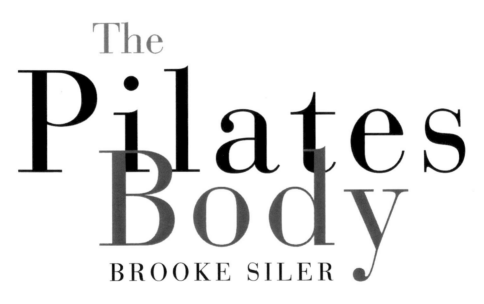

BROOKE SILER

Trainer to the Stars and Certified Instructor in the Pilates Method

MICHAEL JOSEPH
LONDON

MICHAEL JOSEPH

Published by the Penguin Group
Penguin Books Ltd, 80 Strand, London WC2R ORL, England
Penguin Putnam Inc., 375 Hudson Street, New York, New York 10014, USA
Penguin Books Australia Ltd, 250 Camberwell Road,
Camberwell, Victoria 3124, Australia
Penguin Books Canada Ltd, 10 Alcorn Avenue, Toronto, Ontario, Canada M4V 3B2
Penguin Books India (P) Ltd, 11 Community Centre,
Panchsheel Park, New Delhi - 110 017, India
Penguin Books (NZ) Ltd, Cnr Rosedale and Airborne Roads,
Albany, Auckland, New Zealand
Penguin Books (South Africa) (Pty) Ltd, 24 Sturdee Avenue,
Rosebank 2196, South Africa

Penguin Books Ltd, Registered Offices: 80 Strand, London WC2R ORL, England

www.penguin.com

First published in the United States of America by Broadway Books 2000
Published in Great Britain by Michael Joseph 2000
18

Typeset in the United States of America
Printed in Great Britain by Butler & Tanner Ltd, Frome and London

A CIP catalogue record for this book is available from the British Library

ISBN 0-718-14423-6

I dedicate this book to the everlasting spirit of my father, Bern Siler, who taught me about the incredible creative power of the mind, the intricacy of the body, and the overwhelming importance of positive thought.

I would also like to dedicate this book to the tireless effort of Romana Kryzanowska to keep alive the spirit of Joseph Pilates and his work. It is through her enthusiasm and integrity for the Pilates method that we all come to benefit.
She is an inspirational example of the powers of devotion and dedication, and it is an honor to continue to study under her.
Thank you, Romana!

Acknowledgments

The author would like to thank the following for their participation in the production of this book:

Photographer extraordinaire: Marc Royce.

Hair, make-up, and style guru: Bryan Marryshow.

Model dynamos: Julianna Womble, Caitlin Cook, and Dana Eisenstein.

To Romana Kryzanowska, Sari Pace, Sean Gallagher, Elyssa Rosenberg and The Pilates Studio for their superb training.

For the use of their clothing: Capezio, Barishnakov, Danskin, and Norma Kamali.

For their professional support and encouragement: Charles Bergau, Michele Hicks, Kevin Jennings, Erika Morrell, Bruce Lederman, Lauren Marino and the Broadway team, and the entire gang at re:AB. Thank you!

A very special thank you to Debra Goldstein for her never-ending support and enthusiasm! You take literary agenting to a new level!

And to mom . . . for teaching me that I can do whatever I want to do if I put my mind to it! I love you.

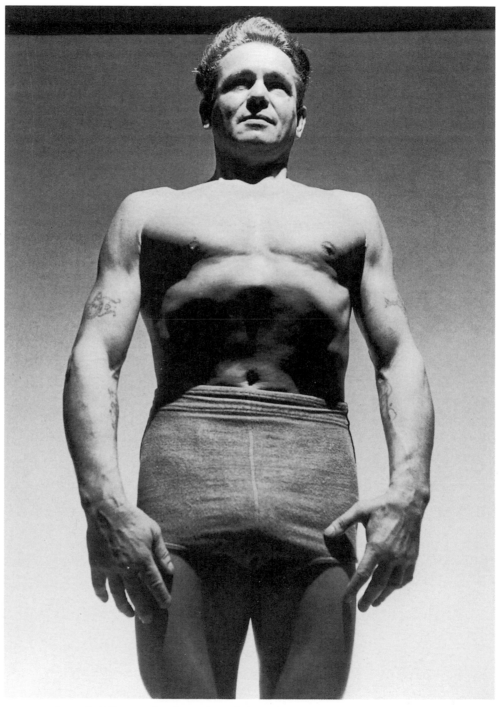

Joseph Pilates, the founder of the Pilates Method of Contrology.

Physical fitness can neither be achieved by wishful thinking
nor outright purchase.

—JOSEPH PILATES

Contents

What Is Pilates?

The Pilates method of body conditioning is a unique system of stretching and strengthening exercises developed over ninety years ago by Joseph H. Pilates. It strengthens and tones muscles, improves posture, provides flexibility and balance, unites body and mind, and creates a more streamlined shape.

At a time when the fitness industry is tripping over itself to create new, innovative trends, the Pilates method, with more than nine decades of success, stands out as a tried-and-true formula of wisdom and unwavering results. Pilates was developed to create a healthy body, a healthy mind, and a healthy life, and people are ready to heed its message of balance.

Whether because of a new consciousness or an intense dissatisfaction with the results of trendy exercise programs, in the past five years there has been a tremendous surge in the mind-body focus movement. People are beginning to realize how inefficient the exercises of the 1980s really were. We may have bought into the no-pain-no-gain mentality, but ultimately that led us to spend too much of our precious spare time chained to the gym. We now realize that while exercise should be an important part of our lives, it should add to and not take away from our enjoyment of a full life. With Pilates, specifically the matwork, we can minimize the amount of time spent in a gym or in front of an exercise video, but maximize the results achieved from a full-body workout. The matwork teaches us that the body is the finest and only tool necessary for achieving physical fitness.

Our old exercise regimes are failing us for another reason: They are based on isolating muscles and working each area of the body individually rather than treating the body as the integrated whole it is. The poor physical condition many of us are in today comes from the imbalance of engaging in complicated, inefficient exercises that isolate certain body parts while neglecting others. If our goal in exercising is to balance our bodies, improve circulation, reduce stress, improve endurance, look better, and feel great, then wouldn't it stand to reason that we should utilize the one method that for over nine decades has proven its ability to achieve all these things?

The Pilates philosophy focuses on training the mind and body to work together toward the goal of overall fitness. Although born in a completely different era, Joseph Pilates understood the physical and mental pressures of a busy schedule. He sought to reeducate us to work our bodies with the efficiency of performing our daily tasks in mind. Pilates believed that his method would propel people to become more productive both mentally and physically. For this reason the Pilates matwork is designed to fit into the physical and time constraints of the individual without diminishing its comprehensive elements.

Pilates began developing his exercise system in Germany in the early 1900s. Plagued by asthma and rickets as a child, Pilates' method sprang from his determination to strengthen his frail and sickly body. He called his method "The Art of Contrology," or muscle control, to highlight his unique approach of using the mind to master the muscles. Interned during the First World War, he taught his method to fellow internees and successfully maintained their health through the deadly influenza epidemic of 1918. During the latter part of the war Pilates served as an orderly in a hospital on the Isle of Man, where he began working with nonambulatory patients. He attached springs to the hospital beds to support the patients' ailing limbs while he worked with them, and he and the doctors noticed that the patients were improving faster.

These spring-based exercises became the basis for the apparatus Pilates would later design to be used in conjunction with the matwork. That is why the Pilates name is often associated with antiquated-looking machines, but the matwork is the original movement system that Joseph Pilates created and is just as effective as the work done on the machines. This book shows the entire matwork sequence and has the advantage of being completely portable. The movements of Pilates matwork need no accoutrements and can be performed anywhere a normal human body can fit comfortably when stretched out at full length.

Joseph set up the first official Pilates Studio® in New York City after immigrating to the United States in 1926. Since its introduction to American culture Pilates has maintained a steady and devout following. It has been the secret of dancers and performers since the late 1920s; Martha Graham and George Balanchine were big fans. In recent years it has been discovered by athletes, models, and actors who say they owe their strong, lithe bodies to the Pilates method.

Joseph Pilates authored a book in 1945 called *Return to Life*. That title epitomizes the very nature of the Pilates method. Through concentrated and creative effort you too will reap the myriad benefits that this unique method of conditioning has to offer, reawakening your body through movement and your mind through conscious thought. The combination results in the extra plus of the Pilates method: a revitalization of spirit that is a crucial factor in maintaining good health and a sound mind and body.

"Ideally, our muscles should obey our will. Reasonably, our will should not be dominated by the reflex actions of our muscles." Joseph Pilates believed in the power of our minds to control our bodies. He proved his theory time and again through years of research and training, and his legacy has been passed down through his students.

I have been involved in health clubs in one form or another since the age of fifteen and have tried all that they have to offer. I spent years as a personal trainer using weights and machines and sincerely believed that I had put all the strength into my body that it might need. I was wrong. What I had done was create a bulky, stiff set of muscles in a young, active body. I spent hours in the gym daily trying to create a feeling of well-being that was eluding me at every turn. I continued to have aches and pains that no amount of training would alleviate, and worst of all . . . I was bored!

And then I discovered the Pilates method of body conditioning. Within a matter of weeks I began to feel the internal strength that I had craved. My movements became more controlled and responsive. I was standing straighter and feeling more energized than ever before. After a few short months my bulky muscles began lengthening and my flexibility increased tenfold. I felt as graceful and lithe as a dancer. Subsequently my aches and pains vanished and I found myself enjoying my activities more. Most important, I felt empowered by my newfound knowledge. I was interested. I was in control. I was hooked.

Two and a half months after discovering Pilates I enrolled in the certification course, and in the years since, I have enveloped myself in the world of Pilates as both student and teacher. I have trained for thousands of hours and

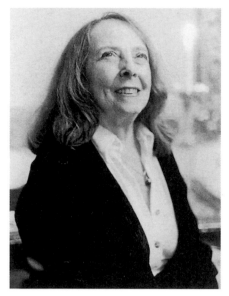

*Master Instructor
Romana Kryzanowska*

have watched the magic of this method unfold before my eyes both in my own work and in the work of my clients.

I continue to study under the master tutelage of Romana Kryzanowska, who was chosen by Joseph and his wife, Clara Pilates, to carry on his work. I bring you *The Pilates Body* in the effort to further expound upon the brilliance of this method in a clear, concise, and creative way. For each movement I have provided visual and verbal cues that will stimulate your mind to action. With patience and perseverance your body will follow, allowing you to experience the efficiency of the Pilates method.

The beauty of Pilates is that once you understand the core of its philosophy, its movements can be translated into any format. Each exercise is an important movement in and of itself and can be used as a way to stretch and move correctly in the course of one's day, but it is not a limited exercise regimen. Many people use the essence of the exercises to enhance other activities; athletes, for example, employ the movements and philosophy of Pilates in their sports. But whether you're an athlete or a couch potato, young and limber or old and inflexible, the Pilates method can and does change the way you relate to your own body and the way you carry it in the world.

The power each of us holds to take control over our own well-being is startling. It begins by becoming aware of our bodies as an integrated part of our creative minds. We were all born with that power. We were all children with active imaginations that continue to live inside us. Sometimes we only need reminding. This book is that reminder. Instead of giving your power away, you will learn to harness it and use it for your very own. This book

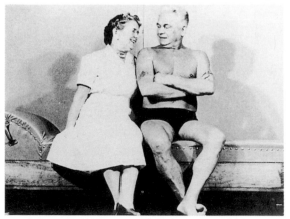

Joseph Pilates and his wife, Clara, on one of the original Pilates apparatus.

will teach you to creatively blend the power of your mind with the movement of your body in a way that is both efficient and extremely enjoyable. It is important that you understand the role you play in all of this. It's all about you. What you put in is what you'll receive, no more and no less.

Remember that with the power of your mind you can bring anything to light, so see your goal and then work to achieve it. This book will serve as a tool to help you along the path, but remember that it is your dedication to yourself that ultimately makes it all possible.

Good luck, and above all else . . . enjoy yourself!

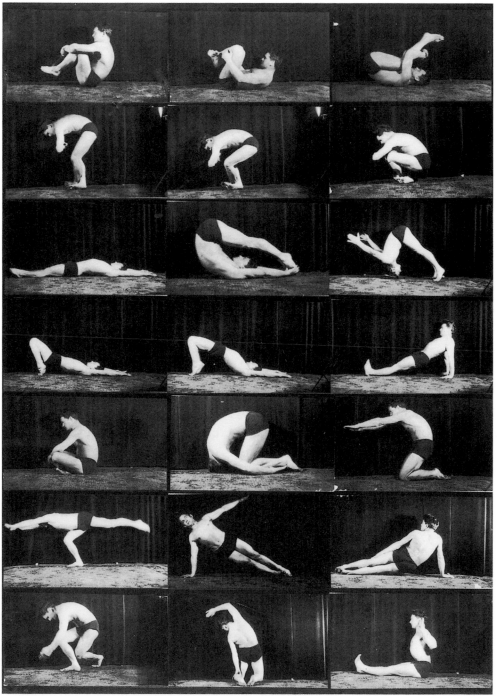

Joseph Pilates demonstrates the "Natural Rejuvination of The Human Body through 'Contrology' Balance of Body and Mind."

Philosophies Behind the Pilates Method of Body Conditioning

"PHYSICAL FITNESS IS THE FIRST REQUISITE OF HAPPINESS"

Joseph Pilates believed that in order to achieve happiness it is imperative to gain mastery of your body. If at the age of thirty you are stiff and out of shape, then you are "old." If at sixty you are supple and strong, then you are "young."

Pilates' development of his method evolved into a vision of an ideal lifestyle, attained only through balance of the physical, mental, and spiritual. Through visualization, physical strengthening and stretching of the body, mental vigor and improved blood flow returns to inactive brain cells. This renewed spirit of thought and movement is the first step toward stress reduction, grace of movement, alacrity, and a greater enjoyment of life.

One of the best examples of this theory is a child at play. The suppleness and vitality of a child are often envied, as if they were traits we no longer possess. Says who? With patience, perseverance, and a strong will all things are possible.

REDUCING STRESS AND FATIGUE

In today's fast-paced life the physical and mental stresses we encounter are dangerous threats to both our health and our happiness. We spend countless hours sitting in front of our computers or bent over our desks, or we're running around, lifting, lugging, and creating havoc in our bodies and minds. Without properly caring for our bodies it is impossible to feel good. Most if not all of our stress and fatigue comes from poor posture, imbalances in the body, and lack of correct breathing. We must first learn to properly strengthen and control our muscles before subjecting them to the rigors of daily living.

These days it seems that only our hobbies and leisure activities keep us relaxed and invigorated, but why should that be so when we can so easily utilize the strength and suppleness inherent in our bodies?

The Pilates method of body conditioning is not an arduous technique that leaves you tired and sore. In fact, quite the opposite is true. By allowing the movements to stretch your body as you simultaneously work on the strengthening elements of the method, you are creating a habit of relaxed effort for your body to follow. We are far too used to straining ourselves in the effort to strengthen our muscles when we should be enjoying the movements themselves.

USING VISUAL IMAGES
TO ENGAGE YOUR MIND AND BODY

Most exercise dropouts claim boredom as their number-one excuse—not hard to believe considering that most people work out only because they feel they "should" and not because it feels good or adds to their mental stimulation.

Think about all the hours you have spent exercising and letting your mind drift away from what you are doing. Instead of watching television or thinking about taxes and baby-sitters, remember what it is you are trying to achieve. Essentially, when you work your body without engaging your mind, you are performing only half a workout. It is the least efficient way to achieve the goals you have set for yourself. The opposite is also true in the lifestyle standards we set for ourselves. By engaging our minds at work without considering the physical toll today's jobs take on our bodies, we are setting ourselves up for a fall. "Sound body, sound mind"—sound advice!

Visual imaging is a relatively new concept in the realm of fitness, but it is by far the most effective. Using visual images to engage the mind is the fastest way to gain access to our complex anatomical system. By using visual metaphors you are able to subconsciously call upon the use of your muscles without needing the technical knowledge of muscles and their functions. If I tell you to "sit up tall as if your head were touching the ceiling," not only are you using your mind's eye to visualize that sensation, but you have also employed myriad muscles you probably never knew existed. You are presenting your mind and body with a challenge that unites their efforts to achieve that goal.

When you create a familiar, albeit imagined, situation within your mind, the body is able to instinctively respond. The creation of that situation is what engages the mind and makes the process more enjoyable. Essentially, it is your own creative ability that will control the actions of your body.

TRIGGERING INSTINCTUAL MUSCLE REACTION THROUGH VISUAL IMAGES

Visual imaging creates a frame of reference for your body to follow. By asking your mind to conjure up images, the innate signaling system of your body is triggered. Like a telephone switchboard, images are routed through your brain and transferred into instinctual movements. Imagine how your body would react if you were punched in the gut. Not pleasant, but the thought alone is enough to trigger a physical response. Similarly, expressions such as "walking on air" or "a spring in your step" can be manifested physically.

The movements of the matwork will become as much second nature as skipping, twisting, reaching, or bending over to pick up a dropped pen. The benefit is that you no longer need to think of movement as belonging only in an exercise class. You will begin to trigger the same awareness in the movements of your daily activities that you have while focused in a class.

Pilates believed that proper movements should become as natural to a person as they are to an animal. When an animal raises itself off the ground, it stretches from its head to its claws to its tail. It leaves nothing out. When we humans move, we tend to focus on one area or another and ignore the rest. The irony is that most everything we do, from walking to sitting up, can and should utilize all our muscles.

Subconscious rhythm is inherent in us all. When we walk, run, gesture, and move in general, we do so without thinking. This is the way it should be, and this is the way the Pilates method was designed to work. By flowing from one movement to the next, you will re-create the natural rhythm of the body. I have made sure to include transitional directions in each exercise so that as you progress you will know how to move smoothly from one exercise to the next.

The goal of the matwork sequence, at any level, is to create a natural flow of movement and then to gradually increase the dynamic, or energy, with which you perform the movements without sacrificing control. Eventually the time it takes to complete your mat sequence should decrease to where you can choose some or all of the exercises and not lose the efficiency with which you perform each one.

MAKING THE CONNECTION BETWEEN PILATES AND YOUR DAILY ACTIVITIES

At first the movements of the matwork may seem unconnected to your daily routine. However, with patience and persistence you will begin to understand how the movements are merely tools to understanding your body. Once learned, muscle control can be applied to any function of physical movement, from walking and running to lifting and carrying.

Structured around the stomach, hips, lower back, and buttocks—the center of the body, or its "powerhouse"—the movements of the Pilates method are instrumental in maintaining good posture and alignment. These are key elements in proper muscle use and make even the most difficult daily tasks seem effortless.

"NEVER DO TEN POUNDS OF EXERCISE FOR A FIVE-POUND MOVEMENT"

If there is one true misconception in exercise, it is the belief that more is more. An attitude such as "This feels like it's really working—let's do a few more sets" is pointless. It's like doubling up on your medication to get better faster. You end up doing more harm than good because you are exhausting your muscles. In a sense, the Pilates method is to exercise what interval training became to aerobics: a more comprehensive way to work your body within the limits of muscular endurance.

The concept of working all the muscles simultaneously but continually switching movements is the most efficient way to build stamina. Because all the muscles of the body are being used simultaneously, and during each and every exercise, there is no need to try to load up on one area.

QUALITY VERSUS QUANTITY

Just because it's not burning doesn't mean it's not working! If I had a nickel for every time I've had to prove that exercise can work without pain, I'd be a very rich woman.

I know that quite a number of exercisers have grown accustomed to the soreness associated with working out and find it rather addictive, but such soreness is not an indication that the workout is actually efficient. Muscle soreness is a direct result of lactic acid buildup in the muscle, improper stretching, or the tearing of muscle tissue. The energy your body needs to expend to repair damage or counteract fatigue is precisely what takes away from the efficiency of the workout.

Pilates was designed to work directly with the deepest muscles in the body, creating a strong core without the pain associated with conventional exercises. And because you stretch your muscles as you strengthen them throughout the sequence of a Pilates workout, there is no fear of being improperly warmed up. There is no ripping of muscle tissue, jarring impact on your joints, or exhaustion of your muscles beyond effectiveness. Each movement has a prescribed maximum number of repetitions. The reason for this is, assuming you are doing the exercise correctly, that you are working your muscles so precisely and efficiently that doing any more is completely unnecessary.

Most exercise techniques focus on the superficial muscles in the body and pump them up for effect. This is fine if bulk is your goal; however, thick, stiff muscles are not necessarily an ideal. For example, the hulking muscle of Arnold Schwarzenegger may be considered attractive by some, but sheer mass inhibits a muscle's ability to move freely. In comparison, the lean and lithe muscles of Bruce Lee are testament to the fact that you can heighten a muscle's efficiency by combining grace of movement with strength.

TAKE BACK YOUR POWER BY BELIEVING YOU CAN

The first and biggest hurdle in exercise is combating the mind's self-deprecation. Many people come to my studio and instinctively begin reciting their shortcomings: "I'm weak," "I'm uncoordinated," "I'm lazy." They are looking to me to fix their bodies, but the truth is that becoming dedicated and succeeding in fitness are already within their control. If you have made the effort to get to an exercise studio or to buy and read this book, then there is already something wonderful stirring inside you. Reward your new desire for change with positive thoughts rather than dwelling on the deficiencies that brought you to this point. Believing in your innate ability to achieve is the key to changing your body.

I am lucky in that I get to watch small miracles happen every day. I have watched the weary become strong, the stiff become flexible, and those suffering from pain become pain-free. There is only one reason this happens, and it is because they have come to believe that they can. There is nothing that we cannot achieve if we put our minds to it, and this is especially true when we are speaking about our own bodies. We spend the majority of our lives trying to influence external forces over which we have little or no control, when the very thing over which we have complete control is literally beneath our own noses.

The many clients that I train on a daily basis all have one thing in common: my constant positive bombardment. Their success comes when they begin believing the positive feedback themselves. Real strength begins in the mind. Stop giving your power away. There is no one who should care more about your success than you do!

COMMITTING TO PHYSICAL AND MENTAL SELF-IMPROVEMENT

In Pilates, as well as in life, there is nothing that will work for you that you do not *make* work for you. There is no good fairy who will come to you in the night and transform your body for you. The physical and mental commitment you must make to achieve your goal is the most important step in the process of change.

Believing in and following the Pilates philosophy will be the closest you come to making a miraculous change in the way you look and feel. Take the time to understand the essence of each exercise and to enjoy the freedom of movement, and in time you will create the results you are looking for.

BREAKING AWAY FROM THE GYM/TRAINER TRAP

As strange as it may sound coming from a personal trainer, I do my best to promote self-sufficiency when it comes to exercise. The Pilates method is an education in body awareness and is meant to provide you with the necessary tools for taking care of yourself. If your gym closes early or your trainer is not available, it is not an excuse to sit home and do nothing.

Autonomy is a powerful tool against the risk of failure in exercise. For this reason the Pilates matwork is designed with the intent of making you the master of your own fitness destiny. Whether you do five or forty-five minutes a day, committing yourself to your body is the key.

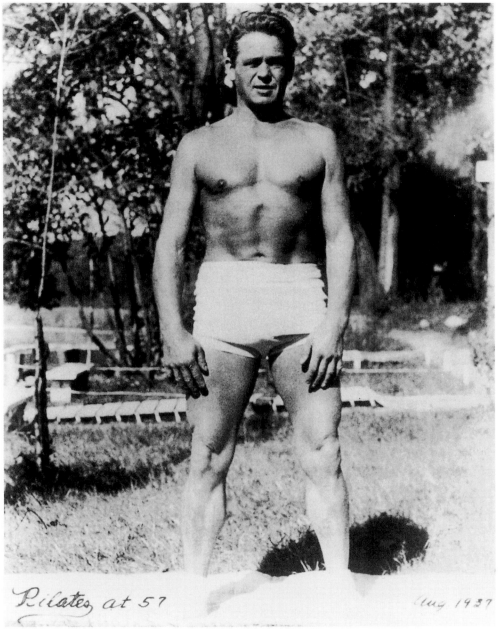

Pilates at 57   Aug 1937

The Matwork Principles

While Pilates draws from many diverse exercise styles running the gamut from Chinese acrobatics to yoga, there are certain inherent ruling principles that bring all these elements together under the Pilates name:

CONCENTRATION

Concentration is the key element to connecting your mind and body. In order to work your body, you must be present with your mind. It is your mind that wills your body into action. Pay attention to the movements you perform and note how your muscles respond to the attention. When you focus on an area, notice how much more you can feel that area working. That's the power of your mind! Use it!

CONTROL

Joseph Pilates built his method on the idea of muscle control. That meant no sloppy, haphazard movements. This is the primary reason injuries occur in other exercise methods. Imagine gymnasts, acrobats, or dancers performing their skills without control. Disastrous! The movements of the matwork are no different. They must be performed with the utmost control to avoid injury and produce positive results. No Pilates exercise is done just for the sake of getting through it. Each movement serves a function, and control is at the core.

INTEGRATION

Integration is the ability to see your body as a comprehensive whole. Each exercise in the matwork employs every muscle from your fingertips to your toes. In the Pilates method you will never isolate certain muscles and neglect others. The very idea of isolation creates an unbalanced body that impedes flexibility, coordination, and balance. Uniformly developed muscles are the key to good posture, suppleness, and natural grace. Through integration you will learn to use every muscle simultaneously to achieve your goal. Your mind is the coach and the muscles of your body are your team. No one sits on the bench!

Key Elements to Mastering the Mat

In order to gain the most from your mat workouts, it is important to understand the key elements that are in play. There are many concepts within the whole that may require a variation of what you have been taught in the past.

Remember that opening your mind to new information is the first step toward achieving your goals.

1. REDEFINING THE BODY

Classically we have thought of the body as two arms, two legs, a torso, and a head. In the matwork the key to understanding the movements comes from imagining the body in its simplest form: the torso. The torso (see Fig. 1) encompasses the space starting from just beneath the skull and continuing down to the bottom of the buttocks. It contains the vertebral column (spine) and all the major organs. The "powerhouse," from where the exercises initiate, is also contained within the torso. By visualizing the body in this form, it is easier to understand the essence of the exercises. Your arms and legs will certainly be working; however, it is important not to focus on the extraneous parts of the body as much as the muscles radiating from the body's core, or powerhouse.

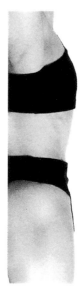

Figure 1

2. YOUR POWERHOUSE

All Pilates exercises initiate from the muscles of the abdominals, lower back, hips, and buttocks (see Fig. 2). The band of muscles that circles the body just under your belt line is termed the "powerhouse." If you think about how you sit and stand, you will probably find that you sink most of your weight into these areas. This not only causes undue stress on the muscles of the lower back, resulting in soreness and promoting poor posture, but also helps create the "gut" and "love handles" that we all strive so hard to combat.

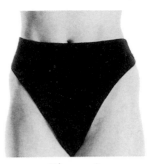

Figure 2

When performing the mat exercises, remember that you should be constantly working from the powerhouse and lifting up and out of this region. Imagine stretching your upper body away from your hips as if you were being cinched in a corset. This action of pulling up and in simultaneously will automatically engage your powerhouse muscles and help protect your lower back.

3. "SCOOPING YOUR BELLY," OR NAVEL TO SPINE

In many exercise methods we are taught to bear down on the abdominal muscles, pushing them outward into a little hill of sorts. The action of this technique builds the muscles outward and tends to push them away from the spinal column. The result of training your muscles in this way is either to develop a slight sway in the lower back that makes it truly difficult to support the lower lumbar region of the back, or to develop a thick middle whereby your back is supported by the mass of contracted muscles that makes having a waistline virtually impossible. When learning the matwork a very different technique is emphasized. You will learn to "scoop" your belly, or press your navel to your spine, thereby using the abdominal muscles to reinforce the paraspinals (muscles that run alongside your spine). This action not only strengthens and stretches the muscles of the lower back considerably but also allows for the creation of a flat abdominal wall. Pressing the navel to the spine

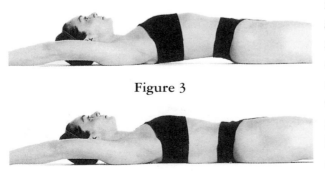

Figure 3

is very often confused with sucking in the stomach, but this is not the case at all. By sucking in your stomach you automatically hold your breath, the very antithesis of the desired effect. Instead think of a weight pressing your belly down to your spine, or an anchor attached to your belly button from the inside and pulling it down through the floor (see Fig. 3). Learn to maintain this feeling while breathing normally, that is, taking in and expelling air from the lungs and not from the belly, as taught in many other techniques.

4. TUCKING UNDER VERSUS LENGTHENING

In Pilates it is key to keep lengthening your muscles as you strengthen them, therefore, any movement that instructs you to "squeeze your buttocks tightly" is not meant to cause you to tuck your bottom under or contract your muscles so strenuously that your bottom curls up off the mat. Ideally, your pelvis and the base of your spine should stay pressed against the mat or be held firmly in position by the surrounding muscles of the powerhouse.

If you are new to Pilates, it may seem difficult for you to begin some of the movements without a slight tuck, and that's okay. Just be aware that your goal is to gain strength and control to be able to lengthen in opposition to your pelvis; in other words, stretch away from it, and keep it stabilized throughout the exercise movements.

5. INTEGRATED ISOLATION

One very important and unique element of the matwork is learning to rethink the point of focus when you perform the movements. It is commonly thought that the areas of the body that are in motion during an exercise are the areas on which the mind should be focused; this is known as "isolating" a particular group of muscles. The problem with this ideology is that it ignores the other areas of the body that are not in motion, creating an unbalanced body. When performing the matwork, however, it is important that every muscle of the body be working simultaneously, since that is the natural inclination of the body and also maintains the body's sense of balance. In order to achieve this goal during the matwork, it is most effective to think of focusing on stabilizing, or anchoring, the area of the body that is *not* in motion. For example, in the Roll-Up (see Fig. 4), by focusing your mind on stabilizing your lower body while your upper body is in motion, the muscles of your entire body are engaged in a symbiotic and highly effective

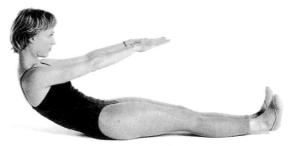

Figure 4

tain a "soft" knee while executing the movements and use the muscles of the inner thighs and buttocks to compensate instead. Throughout most of the exercises, and especially while standing, use the Pilates stance to support your weight. (See Figs. 6 and 7.)

Neck pain is most often due to weak muscles or tightening your shoulders to support that weakness. As you perform the movements of the mat-work remember to stay lifted using the muscles of your abdominal region and not the neck itself. Always lower your head and rest when you feel you are exerting too much effort from your neck. If needed, you can place a small pillow under your neck for support.

9. LENGTHENING YOUR NECK

It is a common mistake in Pilates to tense up in the shoulders as you perform some of the movements. In order to avoid this bad habit, it is important that you think of lengthening the vertebrae just below the skull by pressing the back of your neck toward the mat when lying flat or pressing out through the crown of your head when sitting, standing, or stretching forward. This adjustment will release the muscles of the neck and shoulders and allow you to focus on your powerhouse instead. Think of bringing your chin closer to your chest to achieve this sensation.

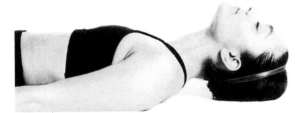

Figure 6

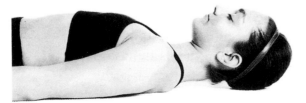

Figure 7

Frequently Asked Questions

WHY THIS FORM OF PILATES?

Over the years Pilates has taken on many different shapes and forms as it has passed from teacher to teacher. Some styles have taken on a genuinely therapeutic approach and are taught in a slower and more deliberate manner. Others have maintained an athletic and more dynamic approach focusing more on movement and rhythm. In its essence Pilates is meant to stretch and strengthen the body in keeping with balance and alignment. Posture, length, and muscle control is at Pilates' core and many different styles of teaching are employed to reach these goals.

There has been much controversy over what can be deemed true Pilates, and in some cases we must agree to disagree. However, Joseph Pilates, in his own books, made it clear that his method was meant to propel us forward to becoming responsible and in control of our bodies and our health. He sought to enlighten, invigorate, and empower us and to that end you must find what works best for you, your lifestyle, and your goals.

Before going into detail about how to use this book to best advantage, I want to address some of the most common questions about the Pilates method.

What is my goal with the matwork?

You are working to re-create your approach to exercise. By using the matwork movements and philosophy, you will create a system that is the most beneficial to your individual body and lifestyle. You are reteaching your body lessons of correct form and movement that will stay with you for a lifetime. Your overall goal is to break bad habits and to connect to and form an alliance

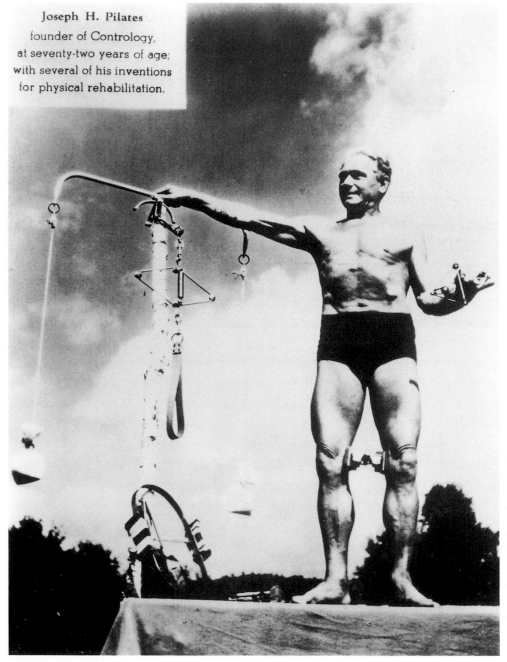

Joseph H. Pilates
founder of Contrology,
at seventy-two years of age;
with several of his inventions
for physical rehabilitation.

with your body. For most this means the enjoyment of moving correctly and reaping the benefits of what that brings: better posture, a strong center, suppleness, alacrity, and a feeling of well-being.

Your exercise goal is individual. In the beginning you should aspire simply to master the beginning exercises of the mat (see "Getting Started" on p. 35) by giving your body the chance to perform them regularly. This takes patience and persistence. Don't give up if you can't get all the movements right away. You are working new muscles, and it will take a little time to accustom your body. Even some of the fittest athletes of our time have had difficulty properly performing these movements!

If you are working to advance to the highest matwork level, then your goal is to hone your routine to where you can add new exercises without sacrificing time. This in no way means that you should speed through what you already have learned to get to something new. You want to move with rhythm and dynamic but without surrendering control. Effort and sweat are sure signs that you are accomplishing your goal, but strain and sloppiness are not!

Each and every exercise lends itself to the importance of the whole. Some of the advanced exercises may not be best suited to your particular body. That's okay. Discover what feels best and perfect what you know. Soon you will find that you don't know how you ever lived without it!

Will I be able to do this if I have not been exercising regularly?

As with any exercise program, it is important to check with a physician before beginning. If you are pregnant, injured, or in any way incapacitated, it is imperative that you get the approval of your doctor first.

However, the Pilates matwork is designed to accommodate any level of fitness. Understanding that the Pilates method is a corrective system of exercise in which you will progress in stages is also key.

You must begin slowly, reading about and visualizing the movements. As you will not have the added benefit of a trainer to correct your form, it is important that you become aware of your body before beginning and throughout your progress. Do not push your body past the point of comfortable movement. These exercises are meant to teach you a new way to *connect* to your body, not to conquer it. Therefore, begin with only a few of the movements; the seven modified beginner exercises are meant to teach you the fundamentals that will apply not only to the rest of the program but also to the way you move in general. Learn them well and you will progress in no time.

What kind of a mat should I use and where?

Any mat or pad that is thick or dense enough to support and protect the delicate vertebrae of your spine will do. A thick carpet or long, folded blanket may also do the trick. As some of the exercises involve rolling back or pressing your spine into the mat, you will want to make sure you are not going to work out on a surface hard enough to bruise or injure your vertebrae. A surface that is too soft is not desirable, either, because it inhibits balance.

The beauty of the Pilates matwork is that it can be done anywhere your body can fit at full length. You need no special accoutrements or equipment to master the principles of this well-designed method.

What should I wear?

Workout clothing (leggings, tank tops, and so on) is the most practical and will allow you to see the muscles you are working, but any comfortable clothing will do. No shoes or sneakers are necessary. Don't wear pants with belt loops or anything that may irritate your back while performing the movements of the matwork.

When is the best time to do the matwork?

Doing the exercises is what's important; it matters less when you do them.

Some people prefer to begin their day with the matwork to wake up, and some use it to relieve stress at the end of their day. Some like it before lunch. And some will do little bits throughout their day. The bottom line is to make sure that you are doing at least some of the movements every day. Try to integrate the principles of the method into your daily schedule and you will find that you increase your strength, awareness, and flexibility faster than you thought imaginable.

It is not recommended that you exercise directly after eating, when you are sick, or if you are overtired. As the movements rely upon the utmost concentration in order to be truly effective, it is important to be clearheaded when doing the exercises. Remember that one well-performed movement is more effective and less destructive than twenty sloppy ones.

How many times a week should I do the matwork and for how long?

Joseph Pilates used to recommend committing to the matwork four times a week for fifteen to thirty minutes at a go. This number will change in stages. Some longtime students of the mat can perform the entire advanced sequence in fifteen minutes and not sacrifice the precision of the movements. The most important element of working with the Pilates method is precision and control; therefore, you must use your common sense to determine your own exercise time frame. In the beginning you may prefer to practice for half an hour. You may be strapped for time and do only five minutes. In either case you must be sure to limit the quantity of exercises to match the quality with which you perform them.

HOW TO USE THIS BOOK

The Pilates Body is laid out in stages so that you can achieve the most possible from an at-home program.

Begin with the basic modified mat (see "Getting Started") and practice until you feel confident in your body's ability to take the next step. From there you can begin building your way up in the full program. Do not try to add too many new exercises at once. Remember, it is the quality with which you perform each exercise that counts!

Remember to read all the instructions thoroughly before beginning. Visualize the movements as you read the descriptions, and then use the photos and visual cues as your reference thereafter. There are always things that get missed the first time around, so periodically come back to the instructions as you progress, and reevaluate your form and knowledge. Have a friend help by checking your positions against the instructions in the book. Or try teaching some of the basic exercises to a friend. Both of these are good ways to stay on top of the learning process. Lastly, try to find a certified Pilates instructor to work with in your area.

Along with step-by-step instructions I have included what I call the "Inside Scoop." The Inside Scoop is essentially a list of tips that I have derived from training hundreds of diverse clients. These tips are meant to aid in the efficiency of understanding the movement as well as being a checkpoint to help you avoid common bad habits. The Inside Scoop is the next best thing to having a trainer on hand, so use its information to become your own personal trainer.

The level of each exercise is clearly indicated, both in the text and in the use of different models.

- Follow Caitlin for all beginner exercises.

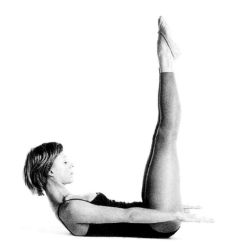

- Begin adding exercises with Dana as you progress to the intermediate level.

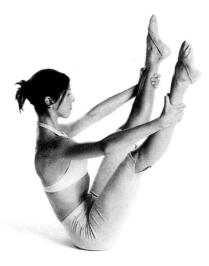

- And follow Julianna as you progress to the advanced exercises.

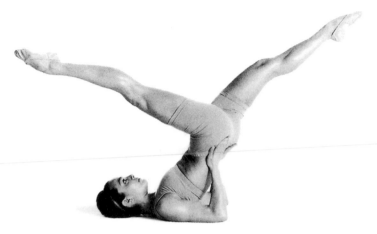

Add one new exercise at a time. Do not rush your progress.

As an added benefit, in each step-by-step description I have included instructions for transitioning from one exercise to the next to create the sequential element that makes the matwork fluid and rhythmic.

Remember that variations and tips on progressing are included throughout the text, so be sure to go back and read over the instructions when you feel ready to move on.

Please note: The models used in this book have been training in the Pilates method for years. Although their bodies may seem to represent an unrealistic ideal for many, they have worked hard to achieve their fitness goals. Above all else, they were chosen for their skill in exemplifying the movements during the long and arduous days of shooting. I hope in earnest that they do not intimidate but inspire.

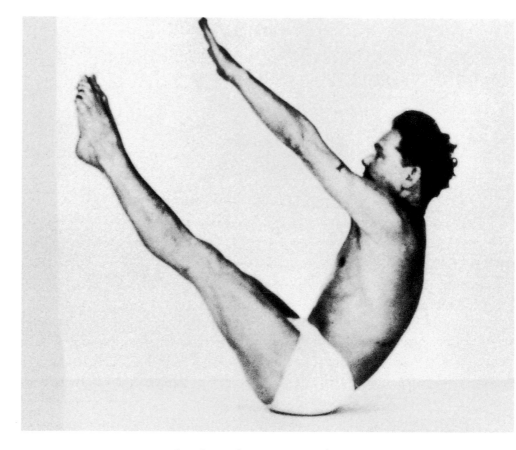

Joseph Pilates demonstrates the "Teaser."

The Matwork

- *Getting Started—Modified Beginner Matwork:* These seven exercises should be your introduction to the mat for the first few weeks, or however long you still feel you are working within your range. Just because they are called beginner exercises does not mean they are easy, so don't be so eager to get on to the advanced stuff. Mastering the beginner matwork is the most challenging part of the program, and once you have done this, you will then be ready to add new exercises.

- *The Pilates Mat—Full Program:* All the exercises, beginner through advanced, are charted with step-by-step instructions, tips for performing the exercises, photos of the exercise movements, and creative visuals illustrating the key focal points of each exercise. Remember to listen to your body when adding a new movement. Nothing should ever hurt when performing the exercises. Take your time, use concentration and control, and enjoy the movements.

- *Advanced Extras:* These six exercises are adapted from the exercises most commonly performed on the apparatus. They are for the advanced student who wishes to add new movements to his/her program. They should be performed with the same caution and control as the rest of the matwork. Just because you are advanced does not mean you are above injuring yourself. Remember to work from your powerhouse and listen to your body.

- *The Standing Arm Series:* This series need not be performed in its entirety. Choose from the variety of exercises in this section to create a balanced addition to your mat workout.

- *The Wall (Cooldown):* The Wall is meant as the cooldown section of the program. Its movements, especially Rolling Down the Wall, can be used throughout the day to stretch and relax the muscles of your back, neck, and shoulders.

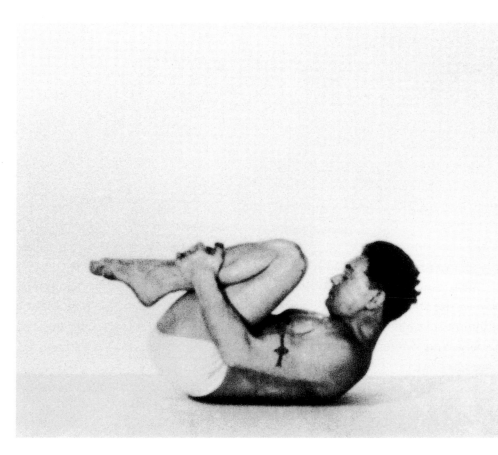

Joseph Pilates demonstrates the "Double Leg Stretch."

Getting Started:
Modified Beginner Matwork

The goal of the modified beginning section is to introduce your body to the movements of the matwork in a safe and effective way. The focus of these seven exercises is on finding the muscles of your powerhouse—abdominals, buttocks, lower back, and hips—and strengthening them to support you through the more complicated movements to come.

Make sure to stay attentive to what you are feeling as you introduce your body to the movements and as you discover new muscles. The modified beginning seven will be the foundation upon which your knowledge, understanding, and power builds, so make your best effort to stay consistent and aware.

Remember to come back to the beginning seven every so often to redefine your progress and get back to the core of the technique. These seven exercises are also great to use when you travel and need a quick fitness fix.

THE HUNDRED

Step by Step

1. Lie on your back with your knees bent in toward your chest. Deeply inhale, and as you exhale feel your chest and belly sinking into the mat beneath you.
2. Keep that *feeling of a weight pressing your torso down into the mat* as you bring your head up to look at your belly button. (Make sure you are folding forward from your upper torso and not your neck.)
3. Lift forward until you feel the bottom of your shoulder blades pressing into the mat beneath you.
4. Stretch your arms out beside you, reaching from deep in the pit of your arm, *as if you were trying to touch the wall across the room with your fingertips.*
5. Begin pumping your arms straight up and down *as if you were slapping water.* (Keep your arms straight and pumping just above the mat.)
6. Inhale for five counts and exhale for five counts, reaching ever forward as you breathe.
7. Maintain this position, pumping your arms and breathing, for as close to one hundred counts as you can manage.
8. End by lowering your head and placing the soles of your feet flat on the mat to prepare for the Roll-Up. . . .

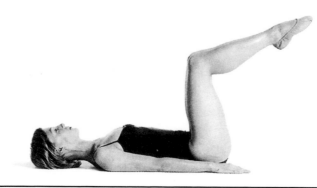

The Hundred is a breathing exercise. It is meant to begin circulating your blood to warm up the body in preparation for the exercises to follow.

The Beginning Scoop

- To stay lifted in your head and chest region for all one hundred breaths. You should be able to maintain a flat back and "scooped" belly throughout.

- Make sure you are always focused on the weight of your belly as it sinks into your spine.
- Keep your shoulders pressing away from your ears to stretch the neck muscles and increase the abdominal focus.
- Squeezing the buttocks and knees together will provide stability for your lower back.

- If your neck hurts, put it down. Do not push to the point of strain.
- Do not push your abdominals out or hold your breath as you go.
- Do not let your thighs rest on your chest as you perform the movements.

- You can place a small pillow or rolled towel under your head to support your neck if it is too difficult to hold lifted.
- Begin with twenty or thirty breaths and gradually increase to one hundred.

- As you progress, allow the exhalations to get longer and longer in order to improve your cardiovascular capacity.
- Begin trying to straighten your legs to the ceiling at a ninety-degree angle as you continue pumping your arms.

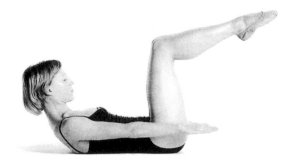

THE ROLL-UP

Step by Step

1. Lie on your back with your knees together and bent and the soles of your feet planted firmly on the mat. Your arms are long by your sides.
2. Squeezing your knees together and tightening your buttocks, inhale and roll up by bringing your chin to your chest and continuing forward.
3. Exhale as you straighten your legs and stretch forward. Keep your navel pulling back into your spine. This is opposition at work!
4. In order to feel the articulation of your spine, it is helpful to imagine this rhythm: Lift your chin to your chest, lift your chest over your ribs, lift your ribs over your belly, lift your belly over your hips, and imagine trying to lift up out of your hips and over your thighs as you stretch forward.
5. Initiate rolling back down by squeezing your buttocks and slightly tucking your tailbone underneath you as you bend your knees. Pull your navel deeper into your spine.
6. Reverse the sequence of the exercise and exhale as you feel each vertebra pressing into the mat beneath you. Keep squeezing your knees together for stability.
7. When the backs of your shoulders touch the mat, lower your head and bring your arms down by your sides.
8. Repeat this sequence three to five times and finish by lying flat on the mat with your arms long by your sides to prepare for Single Leg Circles. . . .

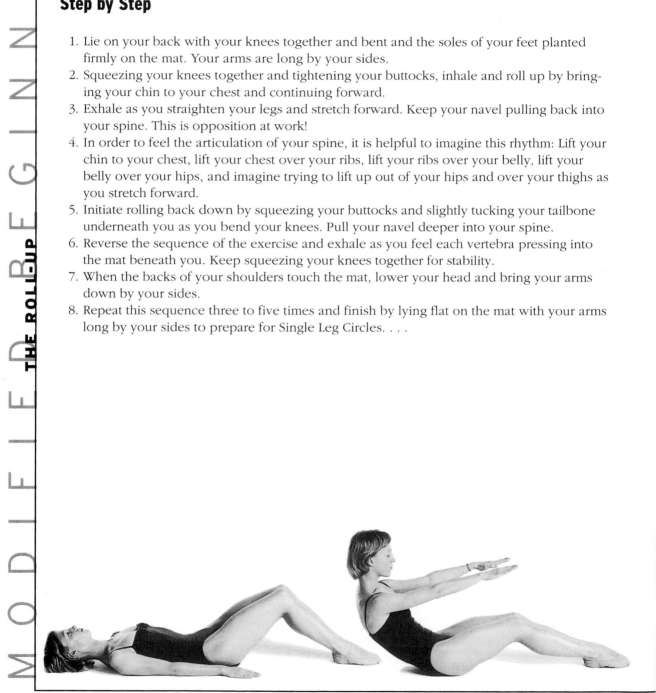

The Roll-Up works the powerhouse and stretches the hamstrings.

The Beginning Scoop

- To engage the muscles of your powerhouse and flow through the movements.

- The key to this exercise is rhythm. Try to feel the fluidity of the sequence.
- Use your breath to help control your movements.
- Remember to squeeze your legs together to keep your lower body still.
- Keep your chin tucked into your chest as you roll up and back down so that you are not pulling from your neck. Think of curling yourself forward, stretching, and then *slowly* uncurling back down to the mat.
- Remember to use the oppositional force of pulling back in your belly as you stretch forward.

- Do not allow your feet to lift off the mat as you roll up and lower yourself back down.
- Do not use your shoulders to pull you up.
- Do not allow your body to flop forward as you stretch.

- If you have trouble rolling up, pull yourself up by placing your hands on the underside of the legs. Remember to still squeeze the legs together for support and pull your navel into your spine. (Make sure your feet are not too close to your buttocks or you will not have the range of motion to be able to come up.)
- Squeeze a ball or small pillow between your ankles to help stabilize your lower body throughout.

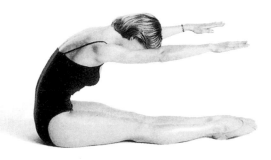

SINGLE LEG STRETCH

Step by Step

1. Lie on your back with your knees pulled into your chest.
2. Grab hold of one shin with both hands and extend your other leg to the ceiling at as close to a ninety-degree angle as you can manage. If your right leg is bent, place your right hand on your ankle and your left hand on your knee.
3. With your elbows extended, lift your head and neck and reach your chin toward your belly.
4. Exhale and watch as your navel sinks deep into your spine. Hold it there *as if you were anchored to the mat below.*
5. Inhale and switch legs and hand positions. Stretch your extended leg long out of your hip and in line with the center of your body.
6. Repeat three sets of the Single Leg Stretch and then pull both knees into your chest to prepare for the Double Leg Stretch. . . .

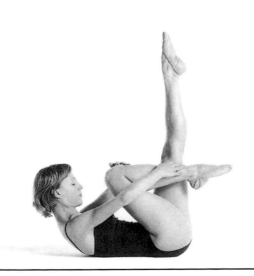

The Single Leg Stretch works your powerhouse and stretches your back and legs.

The Beginning Scoop

- To stay completely still in your upper body as you perform the movements of the legs.

- Remember to stay lifted from your abdominals and the back of your chest area. Scoop your belly at all times and press your spine *further* into the mat as you switch legs.
- Keep your elbows extended and your shoulders pressing down and away from your ears in order to best utilize your abdominals.
- Keep your extended leg at a height that enables you to maintain a flat back.
- Squeezing the buttocks as you extend your leg will help ensure the integrity of the position.

- Do not let your shoulders creep up around your ears.
- Do not lift your head from the neck itself. (If your neck gets tired, rest it back down on the mat and then try again to lift correctly.)
- Do not release your abdominal muscles as you switch legs.

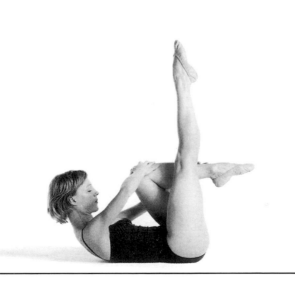

DOUBLE LEG STRETCH

Step by Step

1. Lie on your back with both knees pulled into your chest.
2. Extend your elbows and bring your head and neck up with your chin reaching for your belly.
3. Exhale and watch as your navel sinks deep into your spine.
4. Inhale deeply and stretch your body long, reaching your arms back by your ears and your legs straight up to the ceiling at a ninety-degree angle *as if you were stretching before getting out of bed in the morning.*
5. *Imagine keeping your torso firmly anchored to the mat, as you did in the Single Leg Stretch, and do not allow your head to move from your chest.*
6. As you exhale, draw your knees back into your chest by circling your arms around to meet them.
7. Pull your knees deeply into your chest to increase the emphasis on the exhalation, as if you were squeezing the air out of your lungs.
8. Repeat the sequence five times, remaining still in your torso as you inhale to stretch and exhale to pull.
9. End by pulling both knees into your chest with a deep exhalation and then roll up to sitting to prepare for the Spine Stretch Forward. . . .

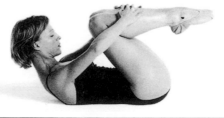

The Double Leg Stretch works the powerhouse and stretches the arms and legs.

The Beginning Scoop

GOAL
- To remain perfectly still in your center, chin into chest, throughout the movements.

FOCUS
- Keep your neck supported by staying completely still in the upper body as you perform the movement. Squeeze your buttocks and inner thighs together tightly as you extend your legs to support your lower back.
- As you inhale and stretch out, make sure your arms are straight and you are reaching in opposition. (Feel as if you are being pulled in two directions with only your abdominals to hold you down on the mat.)

TIP
- If you pull your chest up to your knees very deeply as you exhale and keep your elbows extended, you will feel a nice release stretch in the trapezius region (upper back and neck area). This is generally a very tense spot on most people, so enjoy the release as you exhale.

NO-NO
- Do not let your head fall back as you stretch your arms above your head.

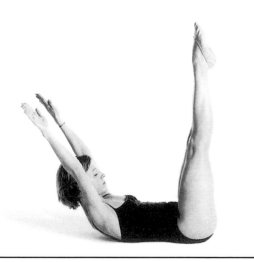

SPINE STRETCH FORWARD

Step by Step

1. Sit up tall with your legs extended on the mat in front of you and open to slightly wider than your hips' width. Bend your knees slightly to release your hamstrings.
2. Straighten your arms out in front of you at shoulder height and flex your feet. Inhale and sit even taller.
3. Bring your chin to your chest and begin rolling down, pressing your navel deep into your spine as you round. *Imagine you are forming the letter C with your body.*
4. Exhale as you stretch your upper body forward, resisting the stretch by pulling back with your abdominals. This is opposition at work again. Your hips should remain still at all times.
5. Inhale as you reverse the motion of the exercise, *rolling up as if constrained by a wall behind you.*
6. Exhale, returning to your tall seated position. Press your shoulders down, and *stretch your back flat up against the imagined wall behind you.*
7. Repeat three times with the goal of increasing the stretch down the spine with each repetition.

Practice these seven modified exercises until you feel ready to move on to the basic exercises of the full mat program. . . .

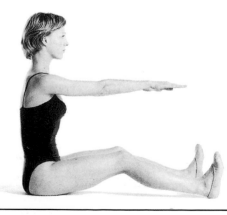

The Spine Stretch Forward works the deep abdominals, articulates the spine, and enhances good posture.

The Beginning Scoop

GOAL
- To keep your hips stable as you stretch your spine.

FOCUS
- Breathing is the key to a good stretch, so do not hold your breath, as this creates more tension in your body and limits your progress.
- Press your shoulders down and away from your ears as you roll yourself back up to release the muscles in the back of your neck. (The crown of your head should be stretching toward the ceiling.)
- As you stretch up to a tall seated position make sure you are initiating from your powerhouse and not lifting your head to come up. (Your head should be the last part up.)

NO-NOS
- Do not let your knees roll inward as you stretch forward. Think of pulling your baby toes back toward you as you stretch.
- Do not flop forward as you stretch. Think of reaching in opposition instead.
- Roll not back but up as you sit tall.

BEGINNING PROGRESSION
- As you progress, try to increase the stretch in your hamstrings by straightening one leg and then the other as you exhale forward.

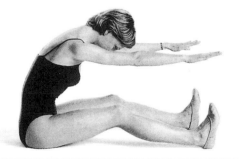

The Pilates Mat:
Full Program

THE EXERCISE SEQUENCE OF THE MAT

Remember that these exercises were developed as a sequence to create a flow of movement. Study this chart and try to visualize the transitions from one exercise to the next.

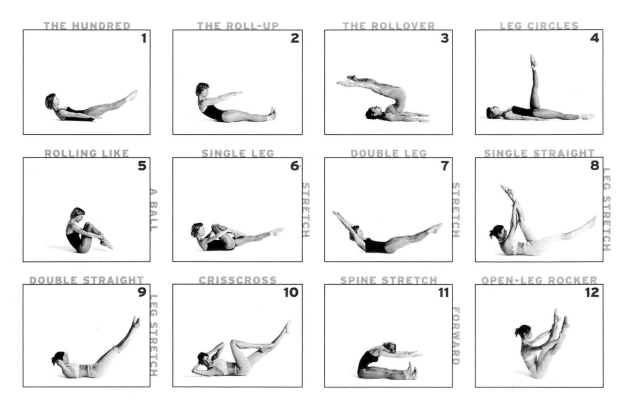

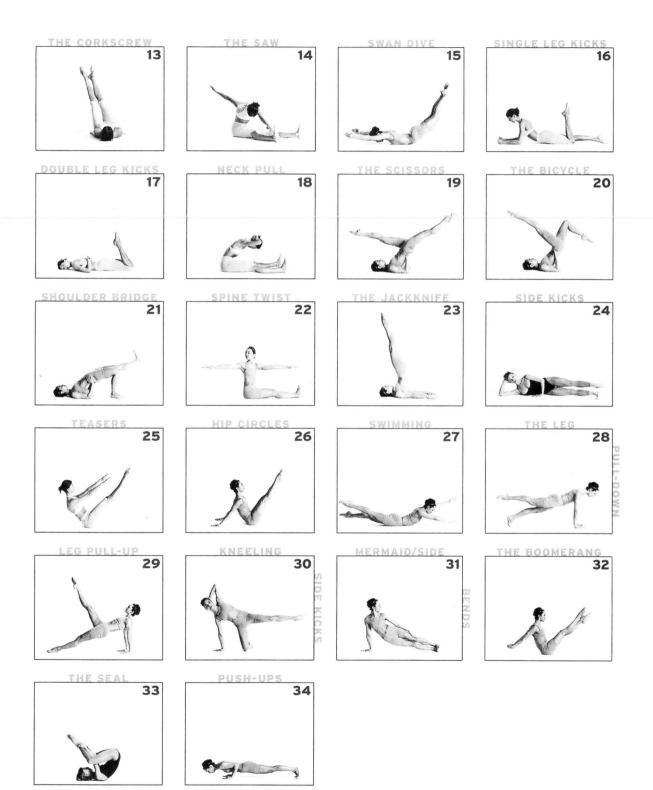

THE CORKSCREW **13**

THE SAW **14**

SWAN DIVE **15**

SINGLE LEG KICKS **16**

DOUBLE LEG KICKS **17**

NECK PULL **18**

THE SCISSORS **19**

THE BICYCLE **20**

SHOULDER BRIDGE **21**

SPINE TWIST **22**

THE JACKKNIFE **23**

SIDE KICKS **24**

TEASERS **25**

HIP CIRCLES **26**

SWIMMING **27**

THE LEG **28** PULL-DOWN

LEG PULL-UP **29**

KNEELING **30** SIDE KICKS

MERMAID/SIDE **31** BENDS

THE BOOMERANG **32**

THE SEAL **33**

PUSH-UPS **34**

51

THE HUNDRED

Step by Step

1. Lie on your back and pull your knees into your chest. Inhale deeply, and as you exhale sink your chest and belly into the mat beneath you.
2. Keep that *feeling of a weight pressing your torso down* as you bring your head up to look at your belly. (Make sure you are folding forward from your upper back and not your neck.)
3. Stretch your arms long by your sides and reach forward until you feel the bottom of your shoulder blades sinking into the mat beneath you.
4. Straighten your legs to the ceiling, squeezing the buttocks and backs of the upper inner thighs together until no light comes through them.
5. *Begin pumping your arms straight up and down as if you were slapping water.* (Keep the movement slightly above the mat and your arms straight.)
6. Inhale for five counts and exhale for five counts, reaching ever forward as you breathe.
7. Lower your legs to a forty-five-degree angle, or to the point just before your spine arches off the mat.
8. Maintain this position, pumping your arms and breathing for one hundred counts.
9. End by lowering your head and bringing your knees back into your chest before stretching yourself out to full length to prepare for the Roll-Up. . . .

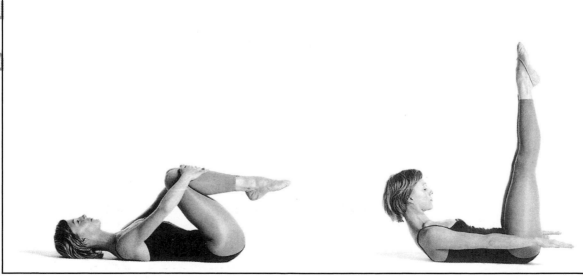

The Hundred is a breathing exercise meant to circulate your blood to warm up the body in preparation for the exercises to follow.

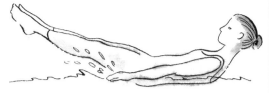

The Inside Scoop

GOAL
- The goal of the Hundred is to be able to maintain a steady, flat back with your feet held at eye level. This is no easy task in the beginning, so do not push yourself to the point of strain.

KEYS
- Make sure you are always focused on the weight of your belly as it sinks into your spine.
- Keep your shoulders pressing away from your ears to stretch the neck muscles and increase the abdominal focus.
- Squeezing the buttocks and backs of the upper inner thighs will provide stability for your lower back.

NO-NO
- Never drop your legs past the point of comfort for your back. You should be able to maintain a flat back and scooped belly throughout.

MODIFICATIONS
- If your lower back begins to hurt, simply bend your knees in toward your chest.
- If your neck hurts, rest it back down on the mat and then try again, making sure you are lifting from the area around the back of your chest and not from the neck itself.

PROGRESSION
- As you progress, allow your exhalations to get longer and longer in order to improve your cardiovascular capacity.

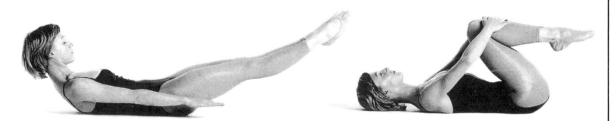

SPINE STRETCH FORWARD

Step by Step

1. Sit tall with your legs extended straight out on the mat in front of you and open to slightly wider than your hips' width.
2. Straighten your arms out in front of you and flex your feet *as if you were pressing your heels into the wall across the room.*
3. Inhale and sit up even taller as if the crown of your head were pressing up and through the ceiling above.
4. Bring your chin to your chest and begin to round down toward your belly, forcing the air out of your lungs. *Imagine you are forming the letter C with your body.*
5. Exhale as you stretch forward, simultaneously pulling in your abdominals. *Imagine you are stretching over a beach ball held between your legs. Squeeze the imaginary ball with your upper inner thighs* as you lift your chest up over the top.
6. Inhale and reverse the motion of the exercise, *rolling up as if constrained by a wall behind you.*
7. Exhale as you return to your tall seated position, pressing your shoulders down and stretching your arms long in front of you. *Really feel your back stretching flat up against the imagined wall behind you.*
8. Repeat three times with the goal of increasing the stretch down the spine with each repetition. End by sitting tall and bending your knees in toward your chest to prepare for the Open-Leg Rocker. . . .

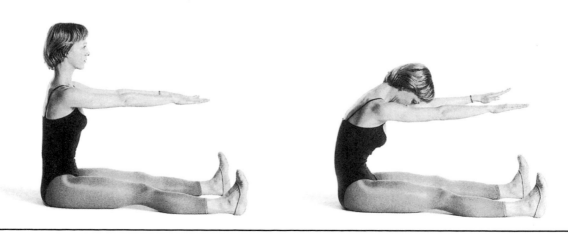

BEGINNER SPINE STRETCH FORWARD

The Spine Stretch Forward articulates the spine and enhances good posture. It also stretches your hamstrings and empties stale air from your lungs.

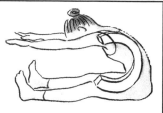

The Inside Scoop

GOAL
- To keep your hips stable and your belly pulling back as you round and stretch forward.

KEYS
- As you roll up to sitting make sure you are lifting from your powerhouse and not initiating from your head. (Your head should be the last part up.)
- Press your shoulders down and away from your ears as you roll yourself up to release the muscles in the back of your neck. Keep the crown of your head stretching toward the ceiling.
- Think of pulling your baby toes back toward you as you stretch forward.
- Breathe through the stretch to control the movement.
- Try to feel as if you are creating space between each vertebra as you roll up.

NO-NOS
- Do not let your knees roll inward as you stretch forward.
- Roll not back but *up* as you return to your tall seated position.
- Do not hold your breath, as this creates more tension in your body and limits your progress.

PROGRESSION
- As you progress try to increase the stretch by pulling deeper into your spine with each repetition.

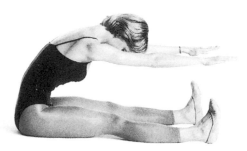

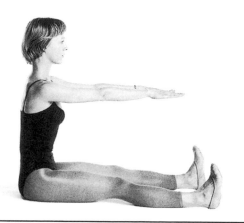

SINGLE LEG KICKS

Step by Step

1. Lie on your stomach, propped up on your elbows, with your navel pulled up into your spine and your pubic bone pressing firmly down into the mat.
2. Squeeze your buttocks and the backs of your upper inner thighs together to support your lower back. Make sure that your elbows are *directly* beneath your shoulders and your chest is lifted so that you do not sink into your shoulders and back of the neck.
3. Your hands can be made into fists and positioned directly in front of your elbows. (If fists are uncomfortable, place your palms facedown on the mat.) Think of lifting your upper body away from the mat by pressing away from the elbows.
4. *Imagine you are being suspended from the ceiling from your belly and must continue to press your elbows and pelvic bone into the mat to stay grounded.*
5. Lengthen your spine and kick your left heel into your left buttock with a double beat.
6. Switch and kick the right heel to the right buttock with a double beat. Straighten the opposite leg when it is not kicking. Do not let it touch the mat in between kicks.
7. Remember to stay lifted in the abdominals by pressing up and away from your elbows.
8. Complete five sets and end by sitting back on your heels to release your lower back. Lie onto your stomach with your face to one side and your hands behind your back to prepare for the Double Leg Kicks. . . .

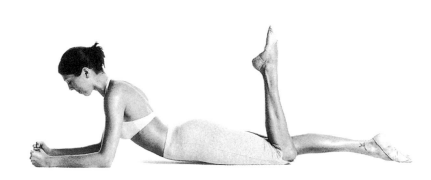

The Single Leg Kicks work your hamstrings, biceps, and triceps while stretching your thighs, knees, and abdominal muscles.

The Inside Scoop

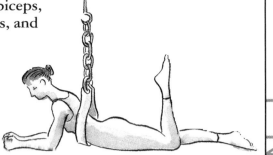

If you have bad knees, leave this exercise out, or simply use the motion of slowly bringing your heel toward your buttock as a stretch over the knee. If you experience pain, stop.

GOAL
- To remain lifted and perfectly still in your torso as you kick your heels into your bottom

KEYS
- The key to this exercise is maintaining a lifted upper body throughout the kicking movement. This is best achieved by lifting your chest up and away from your elbows while still pressing your pubic bone into the mat.
- Make sure to lengthen from the crown of your head to maintain a long neck and to support the weight of your head.
- Keep your upper thighs and knees glued together as you kick to engage the hamstring and buttock muscles.

NO-NOS
- Do not sink into your shoulders or lower back.
- If your lower back hurts, stop. Sit back on your heels and release your back.

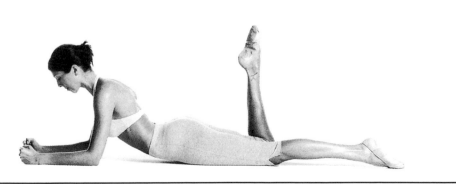

DOUBLE LEG KICKS

Step by Step

1. Lie on your stomach with your face resting on one side. Clasp your hands behind you and place them as high up on your back as is comfortable while still being able to touch the fronts of your shoulders and elbows down to the mat.

2. Squeeze your buttocks and upper inner thighs together and inhale as you kick both heels, *like a fish's tail,* to your bottom three times.

3. As you extend your legs back down to the mat, exhale and stretch your arms back to follow them, bringing your upper back up off the mat in an arched position.

4. Continue to reach your clasped hands long and low behind you, squeezing your shoulder blades together and lengthening your spine. Keep your legs and the tops of your feet pressing down into the mat beneath you as you stretch back.

5. Exhale as you return your upper body to the mat, turning your face to the other side and bringing your hands and heels back to the initial kicking position.

6. *Imagine your hands and feet are connected by a band that is pulled back and forth between them.*

7. Complete three sets of the Double Leg Kicks and then sit back onto your heels to release the lower back. Flip onto your back and lie with your hands behind your head and your legs outstretched on the mat to prepare for the Neck Pull. . . .

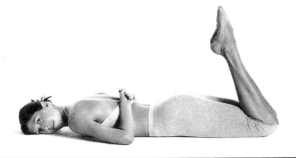

The Double Leg Kicks work the
back of the legs and buttocks and
stretch the shoulders and midback.

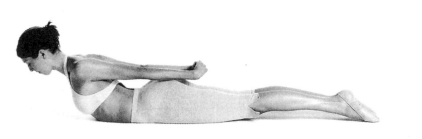

The Inside Scoop

If you have a bad back or shoulders, leave this exercise out.

GOAL
- To be able to touch your heels to your buttocks during the kicks. To press your elbows into the mat with your hands high on your back. To keep your legs together and your feet down when stretching your back.

KEYS
- Make sure to keep your arms reaching long and low behind you. Think of trying to get your hands down past your buttocks.
- Keep the tops of your feet pressing into the mat as you stretch back, engaging the muscles of the buttocks and thighs throughout.
- Make sure you are pulling your navel up into your spine throughout to support your lower back.
- If you feel pain in your back, stop! Sit back onto your heels with your arms outstretched and release your upper and lower back.

NO-NOS
- Do not allow your head to sink back into your shoulders. Lengthen the back of your neck by pressing forward and up from the crown of the head, keeping your chest lifted.
- Do not allow your buttocks to lift up as you kick your heels into them.

NECK PULL

Step by Step

1. Lie on your back with your hands, one on top of the other, behind the base of your head.
2. Extend your legs straight out on the mat and open them to your hips' width. Flex your feet and glue your heels to the mat. Make sure your back is flat and your navel is pressing down into your spine.
3. Inhale and begin rolling up and forward, squeezing your buttocks to initiate the movement. Remember the sequence to rolling up: Lift your chin to your chest, lift your chest up over your ribs, lift your ribs up over your belly, then try to lift your belly up and over your hips. Think of peeling yourself up off the mat and curling forward.
4. *Imagine your legs are strapped to the mat just below your hips.*
5. Exhale as you round your back over your thighs as if taking a bow. Keep your elbows wide and your legs firmly anchored to the mat.
6. Inhale and draw yourself up to a tall seated position *as if pressing up against an imaginary wall behind you.* Remember to lift up and not back.
7. Exhale as you slightly tuck your tailbone underneath you and begin slowly rolling your spine back down to the mat. Try to feel each vertebra stretching down to the mat, as if you were putting a space between each one.
8. Repeat the Neck Pull five times and end by lying on your back with your knees bent in toward your chest to prepare for the Scissors. . . .

NOTE: If you are not advanced, or if you have any sign of a weak back, do not perform the next five exercises. End the Neck Pull instead by lying on your side, and go on to the Side Kick Series (p. 98). . . .

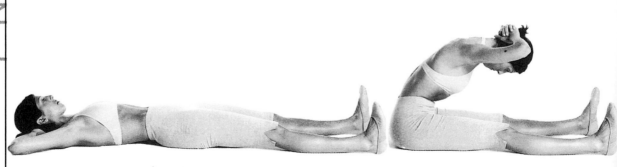

The Neck Pull strengthens your powerhouse,
stretches your hamstrings, articulates your spine,
and improves posture.

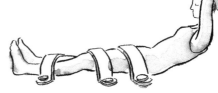

The Inside Scoop

GOAL
- To keep your legs glued to the mat at all times, not letting them slide forward or back.

KEYS
- The key to the Neck Pull is remaining fixed in the lower body as you perform the sequence. *Imagine your feet are two lead weights that cannot be budged. Your legs are the rods that hold them in place.*
- Keep your elbows outstretched throughout the movements.
- Initiate the movements from deep within the abdominals and engage your powerhouse throughout.
- Articulate your spine as you peel yourself off the mat and press each vertebra into the mat on the way down.

NO-NO
- Do not pull forward so hard on your head as to strain the muscles in the back of your neck.

MODIFICATION
- If you are unable to come up with straight legs, bend your knees and use your hands to "walk" up the underside of your thighs. Stretch forward, straightening your legs and placing your hands behind your head. Roll up to a tall seated position and then, bending your knees and replacing your hands on the underside of your thighs, lower yourself back down, pressing each vertebra into the mat as you go.

PROGRESSION
- For an advanced variation, try to keep your upper body more rigid, lengthening as you roll back. Still touch each vertebra down to the mat as you go.

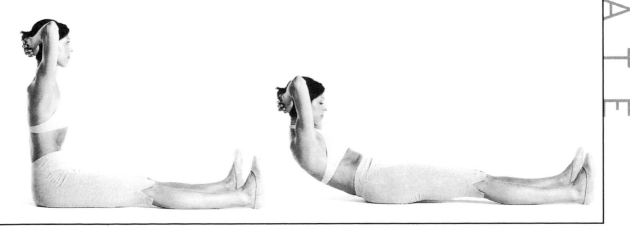

THE SCISSORS

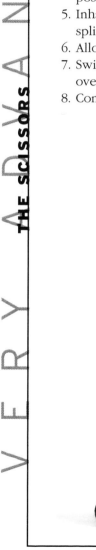

Step by Step

1. Lie flat on your mat with your legs straight and feet long.
2. Bring your legs straight up to a ninety-degree angle, and continue lifting by pressing your hips and legs up to the ceiling.
3. Place your hands on your back, just above your hips, so that you are stabilized in a lifted position.
4. Pull your navel deep into your spine and squeeze your buttocks tightly to secure your position.
5. Inhale and reach one leg long toward the mat while the other reaches over your head in a splitlike movement.
6. Allow your legs to pulse slightly without wobbling in your base.
7. Switch legs by scissoring them past each other and exhale as your opposite leg now pulses overhead.
8. Complete three sets of Scissors and remain in a lifted position to prepare for the Bicycle. . . .

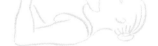

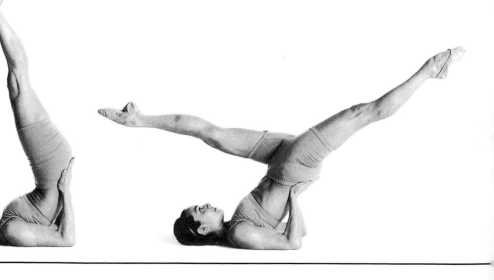

The Scissors stretch your hip flexors, quads, and hamstrings while building strength in the powerhouse and increasing the flexibility of your spine.

The Inside Scoop

Do not perform the Scissors and the Bicycle if you have a bad neck, shoulder, or wrist.

GOAL
- To remain stable and controlled in your hips while allowing your legs to scissor into alternating straight-legged splits.

KEYS
- Keep lifting in your hips.
- Use your buttocks and abdominals to provide the strength necessary for this movement.
- To increase the stretch, think of reaching your ankles as far away from each other as possible as you pulse.
- Focus on the forward leg reaching away from you so that you do not sink into your neck and shoulders.
- Breathe!

NO-NOS
- Do not allow the weight of your body to rest solely on your neck and/or hands.
- Do not allow your knees to bend as you go. Stretch only as far as is possible with straight legs.

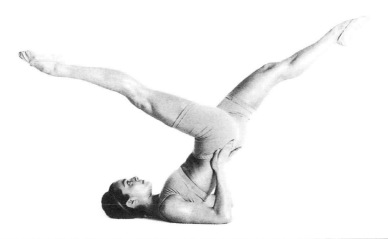

FRONT/BACK

Step by Step

1. Take the Side Kick position (described on p. 98) that best suits your ability.
2. Lift your top leg to hip height and turn it out ever so slightly from the the hip to disengage the thigh.
3. Inhale, pressing your navel deep into your spine.
4. Swing your leg to the front and pulse it twice (like two small kicks) as far forward as it will go without rocking forward in your hips or scrunching in your waist.
5. Exhale as you swing your leg back, reaching for the back corner of the room.
6. *Imagine balancing cups of hot coffee on your shoulder and do not rattle the cups as you go.*
7. Repeat no more than ten times and bring your heels back together to prepare for Up/Down Kicks. . . .

Front/Back Kicks work the back of your hips and buttocks, stretch your hamstrings, and improve balance.

The Inside Scoop

GOAL
- To maintain a long, perfectly stable torso as you swing your leg front and back.

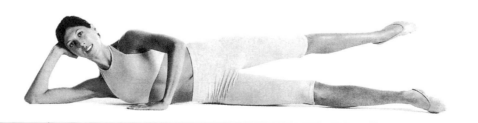

KEYS
- Make sure your legs are long and straight without gripping your muscles.
- Use your powerhouse to stabilize your torso.

NO-NOS
- Do not allow your hips or shoulders to rock back and forth as you go.
- Do not allow your leg to bend completely or you will lose the stability in your hips.
- Do not let your foot or leg drop below the height of your hip as you perform the sequence.

PROGRESSION
- Begin with small kicks front and back and gradually increase your range of motion without wobbling.

TEASER (Preparation I)

Step by Step

1. Lie on your back and place the soles of your feet flat on the mat with your knees and thighs squeezing together. (Your feet should be at a forty-five-degree angle from your knees.)
2. Reach your arms back overhead and stretch your fingertips to the back wall. Maintain a flat back by engaging your powerhouse.
3. Bring your arms forward and allow your head and upper body to begin following them forward and up. *Imagine you are being lifted by a balloon attached to your chest.*
4. Inhaling, roll up to where your abdominals are still engaged and hold yourself there for a count of three.
5. As you exhale, begin rolling your spine back down, pressing each vertebra into the mat as you go.
6. When the back of your head has touched down, begin reaching your arms back over your head and stretch your fingertips to the wall behind you. Maintain a long neck as you do so.
7. Repeat this sequence three times and then go on to Teaser Preparation II. . . .

①

②

This variation is meant to test the strength of your powerhouse before moving on to the full Teasers.

The Inside Scoop

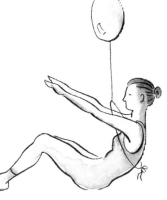

GOAL

- To remain perfectly still in your lower body while rolling up and lowering yourself back down.

KEYS

- Try to focus on lifting up more than forward to keep your powerhouse engaged.
- Keep squeezing your buttocks, inner thighs, and knees together throughout.
- Lengthen as you roll down, keeping your sacrum pressed flat to the mat.

NO-NOS

- Do not allow your feet to move as you roll up.
- Do not rock forward onto your tailbone.

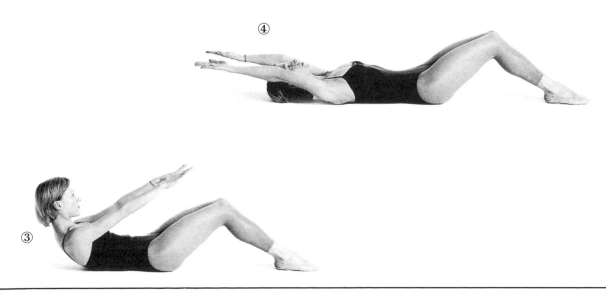

④

③

TEASER I

Step by Step

1. Lie on your back with both legs straight to the ceiling and in the Pilates stance.
2. Stretch your arms long overhead while maintaining a flat back.
3. Lower your legs to a forty-five-degree angle from the floor, pressing your navel deeper into your spine.
4. Inhale and bring your arms from over your head to reach toward your toes.
5. Allow your body to "float" up to your feet by bringing your chin to your chest and "peeling" your upper body off the mat.
6. *Imagine you have a spring attached from your ankles to your chest that pulls you up toward your feet.*
7. Hold that V position, balancing on your tailbone, and then exhale as you begin rolling your spine back down to the mat. *Feel the pull of the spring as you descend in opposition.* Squeeze your buttocks tightly to make sure that your legs remain stationary.
8. When your head has touched down on the mat, stretch your arms out long overhead and repeat the sequence, inhaling as you float up and exhaling as you press each vertebra back into the mat beneath you.
9. Repeat the sequence three times and end by sitting up and placing the soles of your feet on the mat to prepare for the Seal. . . . (p. 140)

NOTE: For the advanced level, end in the lifted V position to prepare for Teaser II. . . .

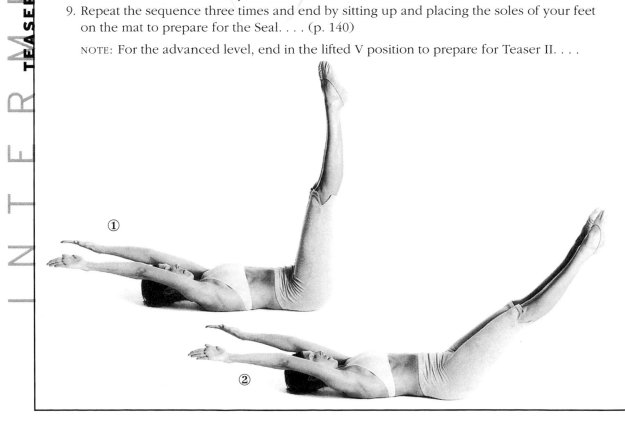

INTERMEDIATE TEASER I

The Teaser I is one of the all-time favorites of the Pilates method. It tests your powerhouse control to the fullest and is a great way to chart your progress.

The Inside Scoop

If your back hurts, stop. Lie back with your knees into your chest to release your lower back.

GOAL

- To remain perfectly still in your lower body as you perform the movements of the Teaser.

KEYS

- The key to the Teaser series is to relax your mind and find your rhythm as you go.
- You must *breathe* during this sequence. If you hold your breath, you will not be using your muscles efficiently.
- Make sure to press your navel down deep into your spine and squeeze your buttocks and backs of the inner thighs to engage your powerhouse.

NO-NOS

- Do not lower your legs past the point of control. If you feel your back beginning to arch off the mat, raise your legs back up toward the ceiling.
- The Teasers consist of very controlled movements. Do not allow yourself to "throw" your body up or drop it back down.

ADVANCED PROGRESSION

- Hold your arms straight to the ceiling, alongside your ears, as you roll down. Try to stretch away from your legs as you go.

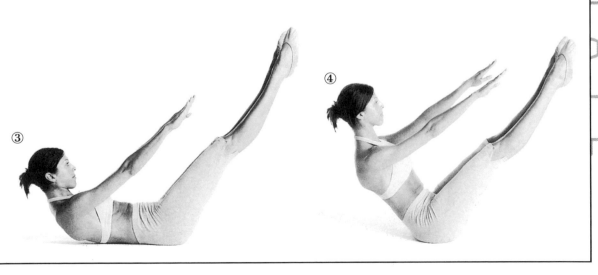

TEASER I

TEASER II

Step by Step

1. You are in the lifted V position of Teaser I, balancing on your tailbone and pressing your navel deep into your spine.
2. Hold your upper body absolutely still as you lower your legs toward the mat.
3. Lower and lift your legs three times, making sure you are working from your powerhouse by keeping your navel pressed to your spine and squeezing your buttocks and inner thighs together tightly.
4. *Imagine your legs are pointed arrows hinged at your hips or suspended by springs, attached to your ankles, and are supported as you pull down on the springs and resist their pull on the way up.*
5. Inhale as you lower your legs and exhale as you return to your V position.
6. End in the lifted V position to prepare for Teaser III. . . .

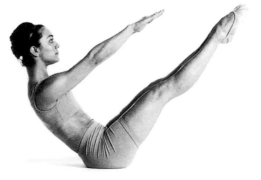

The Teaser II improves balance and coordination and works the powerhouse.

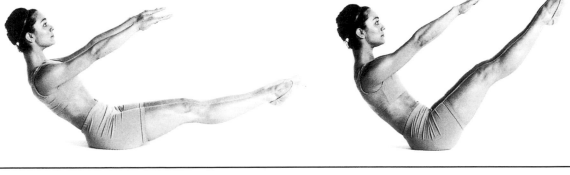

The Inside Scoop

If your back hurts, stop. Lie down and pull your knees to your chest to release your lower back.

GOAL
- To maintain a rigid, lifted upper body as you lower and lift your legs with control.

KEYS
- Make sure you are slightly turned out at the hip and thigh, Pilates stance, to engage the muscles of the inner thighs, hips, and buttocks.
- Keep lifted in your chest as if you were suspended from the ceiling. Think of lifting your legs to your chest as you bring them up each time.
- Press your shoulders down and away from your ears to release the neck and shoulder muscles.
- Total control is key, so make your movements slow and deliberate until you have it mastered.

NO-NOS
- Do not allow yourself to rock forward and back on your tailbone.
- Do not allow your back to arch or sink as you lower your legs. Keep squeezing the backs of your legs and do not lower them past the point of control.
- Do not drop your legs.

HIP CIRCLES

Step by Step

1. Balance on your tailbone with your legs held in the V position of the Teasers, stretch your arms behind you, and place the palms of your hands on the mat behind you.
2. Inhale and move your legs, still held in the Pilates stance, down and around to the right.
3. Exhale and complete the circle, bringing the legs to the left and back up to the starting V position.
4. *Imagine your hands are stuck in cement and you are unable to move your torso except to keep it lifting to the ceiling.*
5. Remember that your upper body is providing the counterbalance as the weight of your legs circles down and around, so you must *press your hands deeper into the cement as your weight shifts.*
6. Switch directions with each circle, inhaling as you begin the circle and exhaling as you complete it. Try to make your legs feel very light as they circle so that you can engage the hip and abdominal muscles and not the muscles of the thigh.
7. Complete three sets of Hip Circles and end by bringing your legs down to the mat and rolling onto your stomach with your arms outstretched in front of you to prepare for Swimming. . . .

The Hip Circles focus on the muscles of the powerhouse and stretch the front of the shoulders, across the chest, and down the arms.

The Inside Scoop

Do not perform this exercise if you have a shoulder injury or a weak back.
If your back hurts, stop. Lie down and pull your knees into your chest to release your lower back.

GOAL
- To maintain a rigid, lifted chest and straight arms as your legs circle.

KEYS
- Think of pressing your chest up and away from the heels of your hands so as not to sink into your neck and back.
- The accent of the circles is on the upswing, so use all the power in your powerhouse to bring your legs back up to the center. Think of trying to bring your straight legs up to your nose.
- Press your shoulders down and away from your ears.
- Maintain a straight back with your ribs pulled in throughout.

NO-NOS
- Do not allow your upper torso to move, or your neck to crane forward.
- Do not drop your legs below your point of control.

MODIFICATION
- Prop yourself up on your elbows if maintaining straight arms is too difficult.

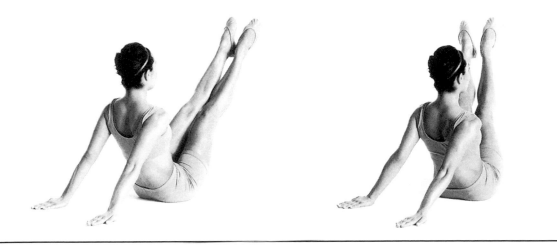

SWIMMING

Step by Step

1. Lie on your stomach, completely outstretched on the mat, with your legs squeezing together behind you in the Pilates stance. Reach your fingertips for the wall in front of you.
2. Inhale, pulling your navel up into your spine as you bring your right arm and your left leg up into the air simultaneously. Hold them there as you lift your head and chest off the mat as well.
3. Switch the arms and legs by lifting your left arm and right leg above the mat.
4. Continue switching pairs until you have a swimming or light splashing motion in effect, inhaling for five counts and exhaling for five counts.
5. *Imagine you are balancing on a rock in the water and need to keep the movements controlled so you don't slip off.*
6. Complete two or three sets of five inhalations/exhalations each, and then sit back on your heels to release your lower back.
7. End by lying on your stomach with your hands placed palms down beneath your shoulders and your legs pressed together to go on to the Leg Pull-Down. . . .

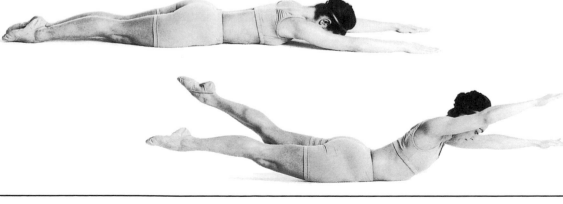

Swimming stretches and
strengthens the muscles
along your spine.

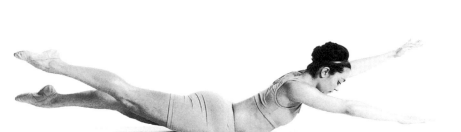

The Inside Scoop

GOAL
- To maintain a firm, lifted center
  throughout the swimming motion.

KEYS
- The key to the Swimming movement is to keep control from your center.
- Use your powerhouse to stay lifted, keeping your line of vision *above the surface of the water.*
- Remember to keep squeezing your buttocks together tightly to protect your lower back
  and to work the backs of your legs.
- Feel that you are stretching in opposition, fingers and toes reaching for the opposing walls
  of the room.
- Lengthen the back of your neck by pressing energy out of the crown of your head.
- Keep your arms and legs as straight as possible throughout the exercise without allowing
  them to touch the mat in between lifts.
- Make sure that your chest and thighs are lifted off the mat throughout.

NO-NOS
- Do not allow your limbs to drop as you perform the swimming motion.
- Do not allow your belly to drop or you will immediately feel this in your lower back!
- Do not allow your neck to crane backward.

KNEELING SIDE KICKS

Step by Step

1. Kneeling on the front edge of your mat, place one palm down on the mat directly under your shoulder and in alignment with your hips, fingers parallel to the mat.
2. Place your other hand behind your head with your elbow to the ceiling.
3. Straighten your top leg out along the mat in line with your body, making sure that your torso is grounded and your center is firm.
4. Lift your outstretched leg up off the mat as close to hip height as you can manage and balance. *Imagine you are suspended from the ceiling by a sling around your waist.*
5. Inhale as you kick your leg to the front wall, making sure you are not breaking in the waist as you go. *Imagine kicking a ball suspended before you.*
6. Exhale and swing your leg back, stretching it as far as you can without rocking in your hips or pushing your belly forward.
7. *Imagine the crown of your head is pressed into a wall and cannot move as you perform the kicking motions.*
8. Complete four sets of kicks on one side and then repeat the sequence balancing on your opposite side.

   NOTE: For an even more advanced challenge, try performing some of the other Side Kick variations from pages 98–115 while balanced in the kneeling position.

9. End by lowering your hip down to the mat and bringing your heels in toward your buttocks. Remain resting on one hand and go on to the Mermaid. . . .

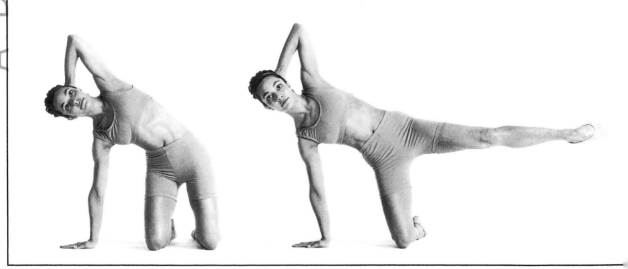

The Kneeling Side Kicks concentrate on the waistline and hips. Emphasis is also on balance and coordination.

The Inside Scoop

If you have a bad knee, leave this exercise out.
The Kneeling Side Kicks are essentially the Side Kicks (pages 98–115) performed balancing on one knee. Use similar images, where helpful, to master the movements.

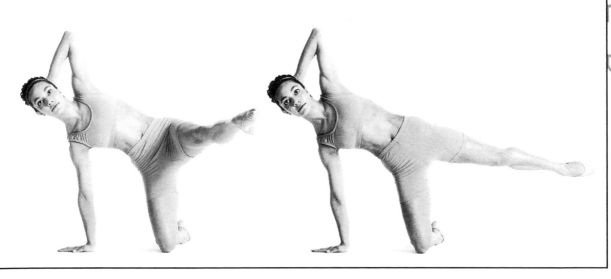

GOAL
- To remain perfectly still and rigid in your upper body as you perform the kicks.

KEYS
- Keep your elbow to the ceiling so that your shoulder and chest remain open throughout the exercise.
- Keep your navel pulled firmly to your spine and your hips still as you go.
- Keep your head lifted and aligned with your spine.

NO-NOS
- Do not sink into your neck or shoulders.

PROGRESSION
- Start with small kicks front and back and concentrate instead on your balance and control before engaging in big movements. Once you are able to remain still in your torso as you kick your leg, begin making the kicks stronger to challenge yourself.

MERMAID/SIDE BENDS

Step by Step

1. Sit on one side with your knees slightly bent and together, your top foot on the mat just in front of the other.
2. Place your hand, palm down and parallel to the mat, directly beneath your shoulder. Allow your top hand to rest on your shin.
3. Press up onto a straight arm and bring your upper foot to rest on top of the other. You should be balanced on your hand and the side of your foot with your body lifted and straight, aligned from head to toe. *Imagine you are suspended at your hips by a sling attached to the ceiling.*
4. Turn your head toward the ceiling and try to bring your chin down to your top shoulder. Stretching your arm and fingertips down toward your feet, exhale slowly and allow for a slight dip in your hips. You should feel a stretch up the underside of your body.
5. Inhale deeply and lift your arm up and straight overhead alongside your ear, reaching as far away from your feet as possible. Allow for a lift in your hips and return your head to a position in line with your spine. You should now feel a stretch along the top side of your body.
6. Repeat the movements three times and then lower your hip to the mat, take hold of your ankles with your top hand, and bring your supporting arm overhead, bending toward your legs to stretch your side in a mermaid pose. Switch to the other side.
7. End by lowering your hips to the mat and then sitting tall with your legs extended out in front of you and your palms resting on the mat by your sides to prepare for the Boomerang. . . .

The Mermaid concentrates on the muscles of the arms, shoulders, and wrists. It also stretches the hips and waistline and helps to develop balance.

The Inside Scoop

If you have a bad wrist or shoulder, leave this exercise out.

GOAL
- To maintain a rigid body and perfect balance throughout.

KEYS
- The key to this exercise is remaining lifted out of your shoulder throughout the movement.
- Stay firm in your center and lifted in your hips.
- Keep the movements slow and controlled to facilitate balance.

NO-NOS
- Do not allow your body weight to sink into your wrist and shoulder.
- Keep your arm directly alongside your ear as you stretch overhead. Do not pitch your body forward as you go.

PROGRESSION
- As this is a difficult postion to maintain, try to map out the motion before pressing up onto your arm. Practice stretching your arm and turning your head while your hips are still resting on the mat. When you feel confident, try just holding the lifted position and balancing there for a breath. Finally, put the movements together to perform the full exercise.

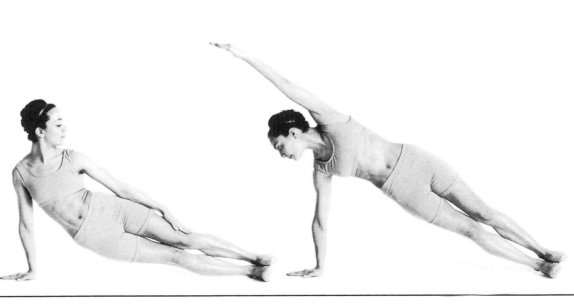

THE BOOMERANG

Step by Step

1. Sit tall with straight legs and cross your right ankle over your left. Press your hands into the mat on either side of your body to help you lift up out of your hips.
2. Inhale and roll back until your legs are overhead. Do not roll onto your neck.
3. Hold this position steady, exhaling as you open and close your legs in a snapping motion, recrossing your ankles, now with the left over right.
4. Inhale and roll up into your V position, bringing your arms forward to your toes.
5. Balancing in this position, bring your arms down and around the sides of your body, clasping them together behind your back and stretching them away from your torso.
6. Slowly, and with great control, exhale and begin leaning forward until your legs touch the mat and your nose is on your knees in a deep bow.
7. Keeping your arms lifted behind you, gently unclasp your hands and circle them forward to your toes.
8. Complete two sets (or four Boomerangs), switching ankles each time. End by sitting up and lifting your bottom forward to your heels to prepare for the Seal.

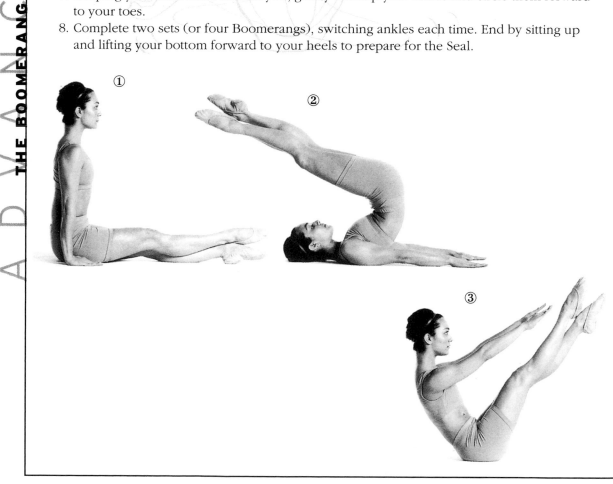

The Boomerang is one of the most comprehensive exercises of the matwork. It stretches and strengthens almost all the muscles of your body.

The Inside Scoop

This exercise can seem intimidating at first, but if you use the imagery from the Rollover and Teasers to help find your focus, you'll get it in no time.

KEYS

- Initiate from your powerhouse, keeping your body stiff so your movements do not get sloppy.
- Keep your arms as straight as possible and push off your palms as you lift your legs.
- Balance your weight on the back of your shoulders as you recross your ankles.
- If you are very flexible in your shoulders, do not lift your arms so high behind you that your shoulders pop. Keep the movements controlled at all times.
- Let your neck relax as you stretch forward over your legs but do not relax so long as to interrupt the dynamic flow of the exercise sequence.

NO-NOS

- Do not roll onto your neck.
- Do not allow your legs to drop down to the mat after balancing in the Teaser position. Think of "floating" forward as you slowly lower your legs and torso with control.

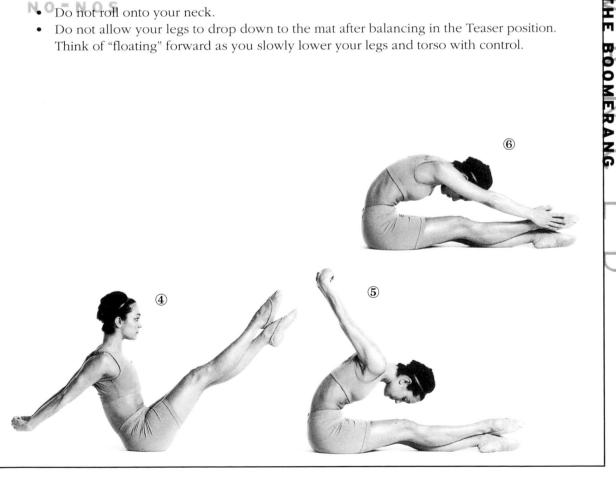

THE SEAL

Step by Step

1. Sit at the front of your mat with your knees bent to your chest and heels together. Open your knees to shoulder width and slide a hand under and around each ankle. Pull your feet up off the mat until you are balancing on your tailbone.

2. Inhale and press your navel deeper into your spine.

3. Roll back, pulling your feet with you. Do not roll too far onto the back of your neck. Balance on the back of the shoulders instead, allowing your legs to extend slightly until your feet are over your head.

4. Balancing in the backward position, clap your heels together three times *like a seal clapping its flippers*.

5. Exhale as you roll forward, tucking your chin into your chest. Pull on your ankles to come up

6. Balance in the forward position and clap your heels together three times.

7. *Imagine you are on rockers, balancing on the edges both front and back and trying not to tip over in either direction.*

8. Repeat the sequence six times, allowing yourself to feel the massage up and down the muscles of your back.

9. For an advanced transitional challenge: Begin building momentum as you are nearing completion of your sixth repetition. Cross your ankles while in the backward position, release your hands, and roll up and forward into a standing position. Use your powerhouse and the dynamic of your arms reaching out in front of you to bring you up.

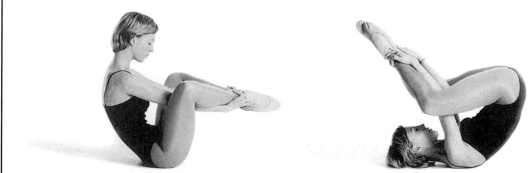

The Seal massages the spinal muscles, works the powerhouse, and tests balance and coordination.

The Inside Scoop

If you have a bad neck, leave this exercise out.

GOAL
- To be able to balance, both back and forward, with your feet only a few inches from the mat in both positions.

KEYS
- The key to the Seal is remembering to relax and enjoy the movement. This exercise is playfully called the "dessert" exercise of the matwork because it feels so good after all the hard work you have done.
- Use the control of your powerhouse and breath to bring you forward and back.
- Allow your legs to straighten slightly as you bring them overhead, but leave your hips down.

NO-NOS
- Do not throw your head back and forth to accomplish the rocking motion of this exercise. Initiate the movements from your powerhouse and use the pulling on your ankles to help build momentum as you begin.
- Do not roll too far onto your neck. You should remain with your weight resting on the back of your shoulders instead.
- This should be a relaxing motion, so do not tense your shoulders or legs as you roll.

MODIFICATION
- If it is too difficult to master the clapping movement of the feet in the backward position, simply leave it out and clap the feet only on the forward balance portion.

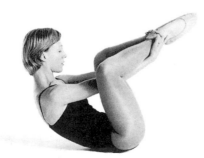
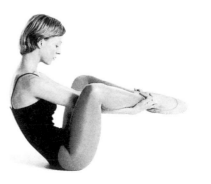

ROWING IV

Step by Step

1. Start by sitting tall with your legs extended in front of you, feet flexed (from your ankles, not your toes) and palms pressing into the mat by your sides.
2. Inhale, pulling your navel deep into your spine, and exhale as you fold your body in half, bringing your head and chest down to your legs.
3. Inhale and slide your hands along the mat past your heels. Keep pressing energy out of the heels.
4. Exhale as you slowly roll up to a sitting position, making sure you are lifting out of your back and waist and not from your shoulders. *Imagine pressing each vertebra into a wall* as you roll up to sitting. Your arms should now be held in midair parallel to your legs.
5. Inhale as you lift your arms up overhead. Stop just before your ears and stretch taller, keeping your feet flexed and pressing long out of your heels.
6. Exhale and open your arms to the sides, pressing your palms downward *as if pressing down on two benches* by your sides. Remember to keep your hands within your peripheral vision as you bring them down to the mat.
7. Inhale and then fold in half, repeating the sequence three to five times.
8. End by sitting tall with your hands drawn into your breastbone to prepare for Rowing I. . . .

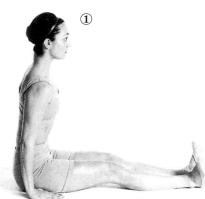
①

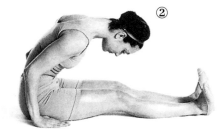
②

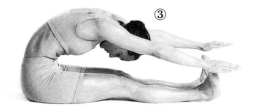
③

This exercise works your powerhouse, stretches your back and hamstrings, and improves posture.

The Extra Scoop

GOAL
- To stay lifted and long in your waist and lower back throughout the arm movements.

KEYS
- Fluidity! Allow yourself to feel the fluid movements as you perform them.
- Press your palms down into the mat as you slide them past your heels to engage your abdominals.
- Keep stretching forward as you roll up. *Imagine you are inflating with air.*
- Stay pitched slightly forward in your hips to keep your powerhouse engaged. Navel to spine!
- Squeeze your buttocks and legs tightly together in the Pilates stance throughout the movements.
- Push your heels away from you as you roll up.

NO-NOS
- Do not roll up from your head or shoulders.
- Do not sit back on your tail as you roll up to a tall seated position.
- Do not lift in your shoulders as you circle your arms overhead.

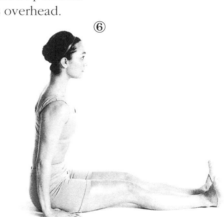

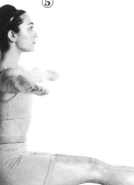

BICEPS CURL I

Step by Step

1. Stand in the Pilates stance with your arms extended straight out in front of you, your hands made into fists with your palms facing the ceiling.
2. Inhale and slowly curl your wrists and forearms in toward your shoulders, *as if you were pulling on two heavy springs attached to the wall in front of you.*
3. Exhale and slowly uncurl your arms to their starting position, *trying to resist the pull of the imagined springs.*
4. Do not allow your elbows to drop as you perform the curling and uncurling movements.
5. Keep your shoulders pressing down and away from your ears.
6. Complete three to five repetitions.

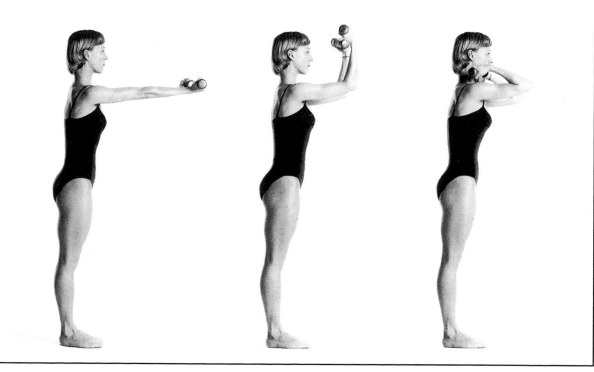

BICEPS CURL II

Step by Step

1. Stand in the Pilates stance with your arms held out to your sides, hands made into fists with your palms facing the ceiling.
2. Make sure that your arms are slightly in front of your shoulders so that your hands are still within your peripheral vision.
3. Inhale, curling your wrists and forearms in toward your shoulders in a slow and controlled motion, *as if you were pulling on heavy pulleys attached to the walls.*
4. Exhale and *resist their pull* as you slowly uncurl your arms back to their starting position.
5. Do not allow your shoulders to lift as you curl your arms in.
6. Make sure that your elbows are aligned with your shoulders throughout the entire movement.
7. Complete three to five repetitions.

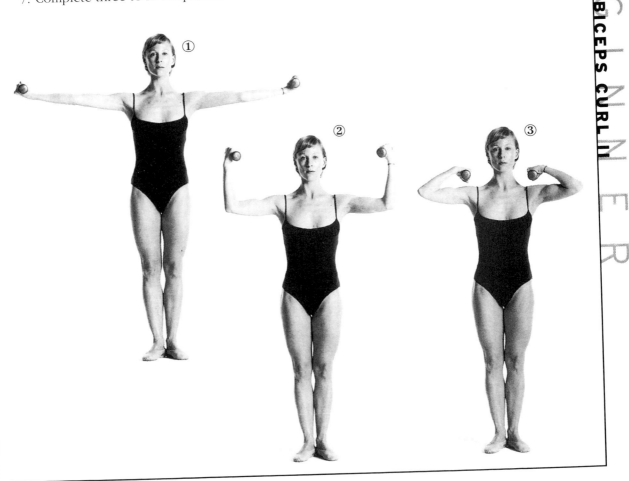

Open University Press
Celtic Court
22 Ballmoor
Buckingham
MK18 1XW

email: enquiries@openup.co.uk
world wide web: www.openup.co.uk

and
325 Chestnut Street
Philadelphia, PA 19106, USA

First Published 1999
Reprinted 1999, 2000, 2001 (twice), 2002 (twice)

A catalogue record of this book is available from the British Library

ISBN 0 335 20067 2 (pb)

Library of Congress Cataloging-in-Publication Data
Teaching and training in post-compulsory education / by Andy Armitage
. . . [et al.].
    p.   cm.
    Includes bibliographical references and index.
    ISBN 0-335-20067-2 (pbk.)
    1. Post-compulsory education–Great Britain. 2. Teaching–Great
Britain. 3. Training–Great Britain. I. Armitage, Andy, 1950–
    LC1039.8.G7T43 1998
    373.238–dc21   98-14516
                                        CIP

Typeset by Graphicraft Ltd, Hong Kong
Printed and bound in Great Britain by Biddles Ltd, www.biddles.co.uk

CONTENTS

ACKNOWLEDGEMENTS

The authors and publisher are grateful to the following: the Council for Awards in Children's Care in Education, Lynda Evans and Christine Rowland for permission to use extracts from NVQ assessment material in Chapter 6; Joanna De Silva and Emma Richards of Orpington College and the Qualifications and Curriculum Authority for work and assessment from the Advanced GNVQ in Leisure and Tourism used in Chapter 6.

The publisher is very grateful to the following universities for permission to reproduce photographs on the cover: UCE Birmingham, University of Brighton, Bristol UWE and Loughborough University.

In addition, the authors would like to thank: Janis Kent at Orpington College; our colleagues at Canterbury Christ Church University College, particularly Sharon Markless and Susie Nelson; our colleagues and many students throughout the Canterbury Christ Church University College Certificate in Education (Post-Compulsory) Consortium, without whose practice and experience this book would not have been possible.

Although this book has been a joint venture by the central team of the Canterbury Christ Church University College Certificate in Education Consortium, individuals took responsibility for the following: Andy Armitage for overall editorial control and Chapters 2 and 6; Robin Bryant for Chapter 5; Richard Dunnill for Chapters 7 and 8; Mandy Hammersley for Chapter 4; Dennis Hayes for Chapter 1; Dennis Hayes and Alan Hudson for Chapter 9; and Shirley Lawes for Chapter 3.

ABBREVIATIONS

AE	adult education
AS	Advanced Supplementary Level
AUT	Association of University Teachers
BEd	Bachelor of Education
BTEC	Business and Technology Education Council
CPVE	Certificate of Pre-vocational Education
CSE	Certificate of Secondary Education
C&G	City & Guilds
CGLI	City & Guilds of London Institute
CATs	colleges of advanced technology
CAL	computer-aided learning
CBL	computer-based learning
CBI	Confederation of British Industry
CLA	Copyright Licensing Authority
CNAA	Council for National Academic Awards
DES	Department of Education and Science
DfE	Department for Education
DfEE	Department for Education and Employment
DoE	Department of Employment
ERA	Education Reform Act
ET	employment training
EHEI	Enterprise in Higher Education Initiative
FTP	file transfer protocol
FAQ	frequently-asked questions
FEDA	Further Education Development Agency
FEFC	Further Education Funding Council
FEU	Further Education Unit

FHE	further and higher education
FE	further education
GCSE	General Certificate of Secondary Education
GNVQ	General National Vocational Qualification
GTC	General Teaching Council
HE	higher education
HEFCE	Higher Education Funding Council for England
IAP	individual action plan
IB	International Baccalaureate
ILB	industry lead body
ITB	Industrial Training Board
IT	information technology
ITT	initial teacher training
IPPR	Institute for Public Policy Research
ISP	Internet service provider
LEA	local education authority
MSC	Manpower Services Commission
NATFHE	National Association of Teachers in Further and Higher Education
NCVQ	National Council for Vocational Qualifications
NCC	National Curriculum Council
NEDO	National Economic Development Office
NETTs	National Education and Training Targets
NIACE	National Institute of Adult and Continuing Education
NVQ	National Vocational Qualification
Ofsted	Office for Standards in Education
OFL	open and flexible learning
OHP	overhead projector
OHT	overhead transparency
OU	Open University
PCE	post-compulsory education
PCET	post-compulsory education and training
PGCE	Postgraduate Certificate of Education
QCA	Qualifications and Curriculum Authority
RBL	resource-based learning
RSA	Royal Society of Arts
SCAA	Schools Curriculum and Assessment Authority
SEAC	School Examinations and Assessment Council
TTA	Teacher Training Agency
TVEI	Technical and Vocational Education Initiative
TDLB	Training and Development Lead Body
TEC	Training and Enterprise Council
TOPS	Training Opportunities Scheme
YOP	Youth Opportunities Programme
YT	Youth Training
YTS	Youth Training Scheme

INTRODUCTION

This book is chiefly a resource for students following the Certificate of Education in post-compulsory education (PCE), or in what may variously be termed 'further education', 'adult and further education' or similar, which all have in common a concern with students post-16. Nationally the Certificate of Education operates as a development of provision such as the City & Guilds (C&G) Further and Adult Education Teachers' Certificate or the Joint Examination Board Teachers' Diploma courses. While directed primarily at Certificate of Education students, this book will also prove useful for students studying these latter courses, as well as for those training to teach in the secondary or FE sectors on PGCE (Postgraduate Certificate of Education) courses. In addition, teachers of post-16 students involved in staff development in schools, sixth-form, tertiary or FE colleges, or in the adult education sector will find this book a helpful resource. The Dearing Report *Higher Education in the Learning Society* (Dearing 1997) is likely to lead to a more systematic approach to professional training in higher education which this book could also support. Finally, the book will be useful in relation to a wide range of development activities for those involved in training in industry and commerce, both in the public and private sectors.

Teaching and Training in Post-compulsory Education is not intended as a textbook to be read from cover to cover. Its purpose is more practical and dynamic. It assumes that its users are both engaged in a programme of training or staff development and that they are either teaching/training or engaged in teaching practice. It makes teachers' professional contexts the focus for their development and each section therefore contains a series of practical tasks which, in all cases, are based on those contexts. However, since the emphasis of courses such as the C&G 730 is on the acquisition of basic teaching skills and we feel the Certificate of Education should build on this foundation by developing the capacities to analyse critically and reflect, the practical tasks are stimulated or complemented by theory, analysis, information, discussion or examples of student work.

Although this book does have a developmental structure (outlined below), users can dip into chapters as they wish. Each chapter is divided into self-contained subsections with their own key issues and can be used separately.

Since PCE tutors teach in such a range of isolated contexts, often with little experience of the sector as a whole, Chapter 1 looks at the breadth of the sector. It questions whether PCE teachers are united by a common concept of professionalism, traces the ideas underpinning some key PCE issues to the work of three educational thinkers and ends with a consideration of the current dominance of vocationalism in PCE. This chapter encourages students to take stock of their own professional/ideological stance which we regard as either an implicit or explicit feature of every teacher's work.

Chapter 2 looks at the central learning processes a Certificate of Education course is likely to involve. Our experience has been that many students have not been engaged in systematic study for many years and the chapter therefore acts as an introduction to the skills required for using such learning processes. It should be particularly valuable at the beginning of a course when students may be arriving from a variety of course types with a range of curriculum models.

With the 'learning society' and 'lifelong learning' at the top of the national political agenda, Chapter 3 considers what this can mean for learning in PCE. The major learning theories are examined to see what they can offer to a sector where breaking down learning barriers is a priority and which is very rapidly moving along the road to learning autonomy.

Chapter 4 focuses on the growing range of teaching skills needed in the increasing variety of roles PCE tutors are being required to play, from instructor, lecturer, coach to counsellor, adviser, enabler, facilitator.

At the same time as giving users a very practical guide to the main teaching and learning resources, Chapter 5 develops Chapter 3's concern with learning autonomy by considering the resource implications of the expansion of information technology (IT) and the increasing reliance on open, flexible, resource-based approaches.

Although Chapter 6 looks closely at competence-based assessment, now dominant in the sector, and offers support to those engaged in assessor awards, it recognizes that the expertise of many in PCE may be limited to such an approach, and so offers a wider view of the basic concepts, principles and practice of assessing students.

Chapters 7 and 8 recognize the increasing importance in PCE of the teacher's capacity not only to reflect on and evaluate the courses they teach but the vital role many may now have to play in designing and developing courses to meet students' changing needs.

Chapter 9 offers a detailed chronology of PCE as a resource for supporting a research-based project students may wish to undertake into an aspect of PCE, drawing on their work related to previous chapters. In addition, a comparative chronology is given for the USA, on the grounds that developments in PCE in both countries have a great deal in common.

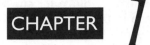

WORKING IN POST-COMPULSORY EDUCATION

1.1 *What is Chapter 1 about?*

This chapter will set out a series of problems and choices which face all teachers and trainers in PCE. Section 1.2 attempts to define what 'post-compulsory education' means and raises the problem of what, if anything, can be understood by talk of teacher professionalism in the ever-expanding PCE sector. The relationship between 'education' and 'training', and 'teaching' and 'training' in PCE is examined, leading us to pose the question: 'teachers' or 'assessors'? Section 1.3 examines the views of three educational philosophers whose ideas are central to thinking about PCE today and invites the post-compulsory teacher to choose a philosophical standpoint. Section 1.4 discusses how 'vocationalism' has come to dominate thinking across the post-compulsory sector and the challenges this poses for the PCE teacher or trainer.

Task 1.1: Preliminary reading

We believe the reader will already know something of the nature and variety of further, higher and adult education, such as:

- the role of government quangos such as the Further Education Funding Council (FEFC) and the Higher Education Funding Council for England (HEFCE);
- the range of qualifications from National Vocational Qualifications (NVQs) and General National Vocational Qualifications (GNVQs) and A levels to NVQ Level 5 awards and higher degrees;

- the role of professional bodies such as the lecturers' union, the National Association of Teachers in Further and Higher Education (NATFHE) and staff development bodies such as the Further Education Development Agency (FEDA).

However, if you are unfamiliar with this field there are a range of introductory books, for example, Vince Hall's (1994) *Further Education in the UK* is a standard work, and Prue Huddleston and Lorna Unwin's (1997) *Teaching and Learning in Further Education* gives basic information in a straightforward way.

1.2 *Professionals?*

KEY ISSUES

PCE implies a notion of professionalism which includes paid employment

This professionalism is a broad notion but one which implies subject expertise

Rationalist thought of the 1960s and 1970s led to theoretical subjects achieving primacy. Does this exclude a great deal of what happens in PCE?

The term PCE is often no more than an alternative for further education (FE). However, this is to forget or ignore the 'training' dimension of PCE, and as a result PCE is sometimes referred to as post-compulsory education and training (PCET). Then there is adult education (AE), further and higher education (FHE), higher education (HE), university education, training in industry and commerce, and informal teaching and training situations. We could attempt to cover all these areas of PCE with the term 'lifelong learning' but this is more of a slogan to be defined than a catch-all. Where do we begin the process of defining PCE? Helena Kennedy starts her report, *Learning Works: Widening Participation in Further Education* with the throwaway definition 'Further Education is everything that does not happen in schools or universities' (Kennedy 1997b: 1). Likewise, we could define PCE as everything that does not happen in schools up to the age of 16. This is a general and not very useful definition. (It is not even true, as it ignores the range of vocational and academic courses provided for 14–19-year-olds in schools and colleges.) The field is obviously vast if we are talking about any learning that takes places outside compulsory schooling, so, as a rule of thumb in this chapter we are talking about learning in which there is normally a 'cash nexus': someone is paying or being paid for the learning that goes on, or someone is being trained to enter paid employment. There are many marginal cases that might be raised in objection. For example: Percy has retired but still teaches his daughter-in-law German in his home; Alan provides a group of interested young students with an introduction to history outside their formal pro-gramme. These unpaid or informal learning sessions do not differ in any way that matters from 'paid' sessions. They are simply imitations of them that become less and less recognizable as they become less formal. This distinction is very crude but it has its point. An idealistic colleague recently declared that she would go on teaching even if she wasn't paid. Advocates of the 'learning society' or 'learning organization' often promote learning, with an evangelical fervour, as the responsibility of all, in a way reminis-cent of the 'de-schoolers' and certain adult educationalists. We will return to these views later. What they represent here is an elementary attack on professionalism. The sort of learning we are talking about is the learning that is brought about by an individual or individuals who see themselves as professional teachers or trainers who are paid for what they do.

> ### Task 1.2: Identifying elements of professionalism in PCE
>
> Do you consider yourself to be a professional? Try to identify what makes you a professional. If you do not describe your role as 'professional', how would you describe it?

Apart from being paid, are there other elements to the professional role within PCE? Such a debate was traditionally concerned with whether teaching was a 'profession' or a 'job'. Issues such as status and salary were crucial. You might have thought of 'professionalism' as a mode of pre-sentation of self or of subject: sharply dressed, perhaps, with a 'PowerPoint' presentation and a study pack for your audience! You could have listed activities in your wider role: serving on committees, undertaking quality audits, designing courses and distance learning packs, recruitment and marketing. Most of this is managerial and administrative work that will often be described as a 'wider' understanding of the professional role. What we want to examine here is a more narrow 'professionalism' which we could describe as 'subject professionalism'.

It might be thought that what 'teaching' and 'training' mean will depend to some extent on what individuals teach and how they go about it. As this book is addressed to a wide audience, we will sketch a general picture to illustrate the problems that this approach would present us with. Con-sider the following typical teaching and training activities:

- a university lecturer giving lectures based on his or her research into 'intelligence';

- a researcher giving seminar papers on her or his research into bullying;
- an adult education tutor teaching A level English literature;
- a further education lecturer teaching GNVQ art and design;
- a practitioner giving talks on his or her research findings in chiropody;
- a lecturer teaching a motor vehicle NVQ;
- a hairdresser teaching trainees within a private scheme;
- a police officer teaching crime-scene management;
- a human resources manager disseminating her or his firm's equal opportunities policy;
- a counsellor teaching post-traumatic stress counselling;
- an instructor teaching social and life skills to adults with learning difficulties.

These teaching and training activities are varieties of 'subject' teaching in a very ordinary sense of the word. But there is another sense in which some are 'practical' subjects and others are 'theoretical' or knowledge-based subjects.

Task 1.3

Review the list of 'subjects' above and divide them into 'practical' and 'theoretical' subjects. Are there any subjects that are difficult to place?

In a paper written in 1965, 'Liberal education and the nature of knowledge', Paul Hirst gave a famous description of liberal education as being 'determined in scope and content by knowledge itself', (Hirst [1965] 1973: 99). He further classified knowledge as follows: '(1) Distinct disciplines or forms of knowledge (subdivisible): mathematics, physical sciences, human sciences, history, religion, literature and the fine arts, philosophy. (2) Fields of Knowledge: theoretical, practical (these may or may not include elements of moral knowledge)' (Hirst [1965] 1973: 105). In this catalogue, if a subject was 'practical' it was not part of a 'liberal education' as defined. This is not to say that it was not of use – the utility of the practical cannot be denied – but it had no logical connection with the forms of human knowledge. Using this description, very few of the activities above would be part of a liberal education. They might be part of a 'general education' but this means something like 'schooling' or 'the college curriculum'.

Task 1.4

Consider the list of teaching sessions given above in the light of Hirst's distinction between 'forms' and 'fields' of knowledge. Do you now look at it differently?

A parallel distinction to that between liberal education and the practical fields of knowledge is that between teaching and training. Making the latter distinction is straightforward if we base it on the former. But it must not be held to undervalue the role of the trainer in society. This would not be a wise move as the teacher and trainer may be the same person in different contexts. Both the teacher and the trainer aim at getting a student or trainee to think or act for themselves. Gilbert Ryle has examined in some depth the differences between teaching and training and notions such as 'drilling' or the formation of 'habits' and 'rote' learning (Ryle 1973: 108–110). When we talk of training we do not mean to reduce it to this limited caricature which, Ryle comments, comes from memories of the nursery. Teaching and training involve teaching and training *how to do something*. They are not 'gate shutting' but 'gate opening' activities (Ryle 1973: 119).

Task 1.5

Do you see yourself as primarily a 'teacher' or a 'trainer'? What would you see as the essential difference between the two?

In the 1960s and early 1970s, educational thought was dominated by rationalist principles. Human beings were characterized by their cognitive capacities. A powerful and positive concept of human rationality dominated educational thought. Judgements about objective truth could be made. Human beliefs, actions and emotions could be guided by reason. Hirst now considers this view to be a 'hard rationalism' (Hirst 1993: 184) and says of his previous position 'I now consider practical knowledge to be more fundamental than theoretical knowledge, the former being basic to any clear grasp of any proper significance of the latter' (1993: 197). Hirst now sees education as primarily concerned with social practices. More specifically, he prioritizes 'personal development by initiation into a complex of specific, substantive social practices with all the knowledge, attitudes, feelings, virtues, skills, dispositions and relationships that it involves' (1993: 197).

Underpinning the rationalism of the 1960s described above, was the thinking of the Enlightenment philosophers of the eighteenth century, such as Newton, Locke, Pascal and Descartes, who established the modern intellectual values such as a belief in knowledge, objective truth, reason, science, progress, experimentation and the universal applicability of these to all of mankind's ability to control nature. This view is challenged by relativists, postmodernists and others who ask 'whose knowledge?', and stress a variety of truths and distrust reason. They further distrust science and the notion of progress and question the damage done by attempting to control nature. They seek to emphasize different and particular views rather than universal 'theories' explaining everything.

Task 1.6

Consider the knowledge content in your subject area. Which of the two views most reflect your view of it?

It can be argued, however, that such challenges to Enlightenment thinking open the door to at least two factors which could seriously undermine the status of knowledge. The first is the introduction of the concept of competence into discussions of education and training. Hyland has made three general criticisms of competence-based education. These are that it is no more than a confused slogan, that it has foundations in behaviourist theories which ignore human understanding, and that there is no coherent account of knowledge in the competence literature (Hyland 1994: Chs 2, 4, 5). Hyland has made some excellent criticisms of various writers on competence as having a crude understanding of know-how, of skill and of the complexities of judgements required in making a knowledge claim. All that is held to be required are certain stipulated outcomes that we can pick out. This is linked with a 'tendency to reduce all talk of knowledge, skills, competence, and the like, to talk about "evidence"' (Hyland 1994: 74). This gives some competence statements a spurious and vague meaning. However it provides us with a very impoverished concept of what it is to 'know' something, that relates only to the performance of work functions.

Task 1.7

Competence and knowledge: find examples of competence statements from your own or another subject, or from a teacher training course. Consider what concept of knowledge they embody, and see if it makes sense. Do they refer to narrow skills or dispositions or to broad general capacities? Do they adequately take account of the nature of judgement? You might like to review Hyland's criticisms (1994: Chs 5, 8) and how far the introduction of GNVQs has gone to meet them.

There is a hint of paradox in that competence-based training schemes are often couched in the empowering 'student-centred' language of progressive or humanistic education. But by emphasizing learning by doing, rather than becoming critical thinkers, competence-based programmes require students to be both intellectually passive and yet very busy. Keeping students working at gathering evidence to establish competence seems to many critics to be the introduction of the discipline of the workplace in the interest of the employer.

Task 1.8

To what extent have you observed the conjunction of competence-based training programmes and humanistic or student-centred philosophies? Try to find a clear example of such a conjunction in a course document or handbook.

The second way in which knowledge could be seen to be devalued concerns the introduction of competence-based programmes of teacher training. The absence of theory and academic knowledge in teacher training programmes is a result of many years of government spokespeople blaming theory, particularly that of the 1960s, for all the problems in education, if not all the ills of society! It is hardly surprising, therefore, that we find competence-based schemes predominating in teacher education. In FE the early 1990s saw the introduction of the competence-based vocational assessor qualifications (D32 and D33) by the Training and Development Lead Body (TDLB), the launch of a competence-based C&G Further and Adult Education Teacher's Certificate and the start of many competence-based Certificate in Education (FE) courses. The outcome of many of these courses could be said to be the deprofessionalization of the post-compulsory teacher (Hyland 1994: 93). The replication in teacher training, at all levels, of the competence-based model means that the model of control applied to students could also operate with staff. It would be a work-related, operational form of discipline that would be adopted, but it would be self-imposed. Many staff in PCE will have obtained D32 and D33 and other competence-based qualifications. Despite some early cynicism, these programmes are now universally accepted. Teachers and trainers in AE and FE have come to see themselves as assessors, checking portfolios to see if there is evidence that student learning has occurred. It is difficult to find ways of opposing these schemes when not only your own subject knowledge, but academic knowledge itself is being challenged. There is a danger of this view spreading to HE through the implementation of the Dearing Report *Higher Education in the Learning Society* (Dearing 1997). Dearing proposes to make teacher training compulsory for all new staff in HE and to establish a national institute for learning and teaching in HE. The most likely outcome of this will be a competence-based scheme similar to those found in FE. The crucial difference here is that the business of HE is knowledge and research, not competence or skills. It is the ethos created by this which is what makes teaching so exciting for many at this level. Dearing's proposals to make HE teaching more learner-centred will not necessarily help students. The idea is that the student is not to be passive but must actively engage in learning. But, crucially, Dearing's general view of knowledge is as a commodity that can be delivered by teachers or through IT. This could reduce all teachers in HE to the position that many FE teachers now find themselves in: as assessors checking off whether we have evidence that learning has occurred. The engagement and interaction with research-based knowledge could become a rare experience.

Task 1.9: Teaching or assessing?

The argument we have put forward is that there is a danger that in devaluing knowledge and critical thinking, we necessarily turn from being teachers to being assessors. Consider whether this is true by reflecting upon how much of your own teaching involves imparting knowledge and developing critical thinking.

It may be thought that the notion of the post-compulsory teacher or trainer as a 'reflective practitioner' could be a way out of the teacher or assessor dilemma. There are problems in understanding what the phrase 'reflective practitioner' means to most people and even of making sense of the most careful expositions (see Gilroy 1993). The term appears to replicate the use of humanistic, student-centred rationales for competence-based programmes for students and trainees. It confines the teacher or trainer to their particular concerns in the classroom and redefines 'theory' to mean the systematic restructuring of the teacher's own experience and ideas. In this way, the model rejects a rationalist model of objective truth (see Elliott 1993). In the context of a general attack on academic knowledge and critical thinking, the term 'reflective practitioner' might not, as we may be tempted to think, allow us to subvert the competence-based curriculum. The theorists of reflective practice could be involved in an implicit attack on just this possibility, however much they dislike the competence-based approach.

Task 1.10

Which model(s) of teacher education does your Certificate of Education course presuppose? Do you consider any of the dangers of competence-based or reflective practitioner approaches outlined above have the potential to affect you?

1.3   *Three educational thinkers*

We may never think to formulate our educational philosophy, but the terms in which we describe our professional practice will nevertheless indicate a leaning towards some form of articulated philosophy. Our argument is that we all have a 'philosophical style' as much as we have a 'teaching and learning style'.

Task 1.11: Identifying your educational philosophy

Consider the three groups of ideas below and select that which best describes your idea of what education should be about.

1 Critical thinking, the development of knowledge, the search for objective truth, with the teacher having authority about these matters (Socrates).
2 Personal development, autonomy in learning, growth to reach natural potential, the teacher is the facilitator of learning (Rousseau).
3 Knowledge should be useful, socially relevant, involve problem solving and be taught through practical activities; teaching should be cooperative and democratic (Dewey).

Each of these sets of ideas reflect the views of one of the philosophers we discuss below. You might have found it difficult to choose just one view and this is understandable but, in the end, we argue that they are largely *incompatible*. Review your choice after reading this section.

Socrates, Rousseau and Dewey have been chosen because there is still heated debate today about whether their influence on education, and PCE in particular, has been positive or negative. This may seem to be an eccentric claim as only one (Dewey) features explicitly in many discussions of post-compulsory education and training. Rousseau appears implicitly in some adult education theories, while Socrates – now as in the Athens of 399BC – is accused of corrupting the minds of youth with his ideas.

Socrates

Socrates (469–399BC): Athenian philosopher, whose ideas come to us from Plato (429–347BC). In 387BC Plato founded a school in a grove in Athens that became known as the 'Academy', which existed for over 900 years. Plato's major educational works are the *Republic* (366BC) and the *Meno* (387BC). Another work referred to below, the *Apology*, was written in the decade after Socrates' death

'The Socratic education begins . . . with the awakening of the mind to the need for criticism, to the uncertainty of the principles by which it supposed itself to be guided' (Anderson 1980a: 69). Criticism is at the heart of the Socratic philosophical method, but it is a criticism that seeks to show that wisdom is 'not thinking that you know what you do not know'. Socrates is wise to the extent that he does not claim to have knowledge but nevertheless seeks knowledge by a ruthless examination of the claims of individuals to have knowledge or wisdom. It is not an empirical method proceeding by reference to facts but a rationalist approach that works through the exposure of contradictions and absurdities in someone's thinking. This method can be irritating for the modern reader of the Platonic dialogues who sees his or her opinions and beliefs subjected to it (Buchanan 1982: 21). Something of the impact of this method on individuals can be gleaned from Socrates' cross-examination of Meletus at his trial, recounted in the *Apology*. Here Meletus is forced into a contradiction by being made to claim that Socrates believes in no gods and yet to see that his charge against Socrates could only be made against someone who believed in gods (Plato, *Apology*: 37–67). This is a method of teaching through which the teacher reveals a person's ignorance to them through the dialectic of discussion and the questioning of answers. Although there is debate about this, the term 'philosophy' originally meant not 'love of wisdom' but 'love of a wise friend'. It is a wise teacher who shows you your ignorance and education thus requires a teacher to be in an entirely superior position to the pupil. An example of this method is given in the celebrated passages in the *Meno* (Plato, *Meno*: 82a–85e) where Socrates questions a slave boy about geometry. He elicits from him the recollection that the square of the area of a square is equal to its diagonal. The slave boy responds confidently to the early questions but ultimately recognizes his ignorance 'It's no use Socrates, I just don't know' (p. 84a). This 'numbing' and 'perplexing' part of the Socratic process, or the *elenchus*, does away with false knowledge and instils the desire to learn. We are not concerned here with this proof of the theory of anamnesis, or the remembering of the immortal soul in its contemporary state, but with Socrates' methodology. For Socrates, unlike Plato, there is no end to the process of critical questioning.

It is a common mistake to confuse the views of Plato and Socrates because almost all of what we know of Socrates' teaching comes from Plato's dialogues. Some commentators make excellent distinctions between the two thinkers (Holland 1980: 18; Perkinson 1980: 14–30; Tarrant 1993: xv–xxii). We will only make the broad distinction that for Socrates education was solely about learning to be critical whereas for Plato education led, by the process of criticism, to truth. The view that education is fundamentally about criticism, however, does not require us to accept the Socratic view of wisdom nor the metaphysic of Platonism.

Most discussions of the Socratic idea of education in colleges and in educational textbooks look at the system of schooling set out in the *Republic*, ignoring the discussion of the dialectic in Book VII (Plato, *Republic*: 546–84) and in the earlier dialogues. This gives undue emphasis to what Plato would consider the lower processes of education, which are really forms of training and habit formation (see Holland 1980: 18–21). In our short discussion we have tried to give an indication of the power and value of what is now dismissed by the proponents of reflective practice as 'theory-based and impractical' rationalism (Elliott 1993: 1).

In summary, the Socratic education is about the need for criticism. To overcome ignorance it utilizes a certain method: the dialectic of questioning and testing ideas. In turn, this demands that the teacher guide the pupil through a process of learning to be critical which may be perplexing and numbing. Finally, the process may or may not lead to knowledge in the form of objective truth, but that is always the goal.

> **Task 1.12: Education as critical thinking**
>
> Is the development of critical thinking at the heart of your concept of education? If not, what role has criticism in your idea of education? Consider how important the element of critical thinking is in your particular subject area. If you are a trainer, are there ways in which you encourage a critical approach?
>
> *Further reading*: Plato's works are accessible and easy to read. The *Apology* and *Meno* are good starting points. Both are short and relevant to contemporary educational debates about the role of the teacher. There are many editions but it is an advantage to have one with a commentary.

Rousseau

Jean Jacques Rousseau (1712–78): essayist and philosopher of the Enlightenment period. Major educational work: *Émile* (1762).

Rousseau is a thinker of the Enlightenment period but stands in romantic reaction to it. In Section 1.2 we have already considered criticism of the Enlightenment tradition, but it may be helpful to state once again the basic principle of the Enlightenment as: a belief in the universal applicability and value to humanity in overcoming our dependence on nature by means of science, reason, progress, and experimentation. Rousseau's work is not aimed at defending the *ancien régime*. He believes in the revolution that is sweeping it away but is concerned at what it is creating, the new enemy, the 'bourgeois'. He is a man who thinks only of himself and whose prime motivation is fear of his own death (Bloom 1991: 3–28). Rousseau's model of the bourgeois is based upon the pre-revolutionary bourgeois he saw growing up around him in France but also on the English gentleman whose education is described in John Locke's ([1693] 1989) *Some Thoughts Concerning Education*.

It is surprising that Rousseau has not been adopted as the educational thinker of the so-called 'postmodern age' or of 'new age thinking'. *Émile* begins with the declaration: 'Everything is good as it leaves the hands of the Author of things; everything degenerates in the hands of man' (Rousseau [1762] 1991: 37). Society, even living in small groups, corrupts man's nature. It is to nature that we must turn to save us from disfiguring everything. Rousseau describes the child as a plant, and organic and growth metaphors abound. 'Plants are shaped by cultivation, and men by education' (p. 38).

Rousseau uses a wide definition of education to mean any change brought about after our birth. It is, therefore, threefold and comes from nature, men and things. It is only the education by men that we have entire control of so we must use it to ensure that education from nature is the dominant form. Nature is defined as a state in which our dispositions are uncorrupted by opinion (Rousseau [1762] 1991: 39). Rousseau enjoins

mothers to 'Observe nature and follow the path it maps out for you' (p. 41). In thinking to correct or change that path we do more harm than good.

Man in his natural state is entirely for himself. Both Locke and Rousseau held this opinion. In Locke's view the adult knows best and denies the child all his wants while giving reasons that are appropriate to the age of the child (Locke [1693] 1989: Sections 39 and 44). The adult dominates and only looks for the man in the child. But Locke seeks to limit impositions and restrictions on freedom only to those that are absolutely necessary. Rousseau believes that if a child is educated by nature and things as described in the story of Émile's education, he will come to accept restrictions as legitimate rather than necessary. He will then impose them on himself. This is the essence of the good citizen. Of course, adults are active in the education of the child but only to ensure that nature takes its course. The child or young person must find out for themselves but their tutor arranges things so that certain results will follow.

In the natural order, all men are equal (Rousseau [1762] 1991: 41) so he considers only the education of the individual into man's estate. Although Rousseau was a primitivist to a certain extent, he wants men to live in society and not return to the condition of some mythical 'noble savage'. He praises Plato's *Republic* as 'the most beautiful educational treatise ever written' ([1762] 1991: 40). Yet he believes its vision of public education can no longer exist. His concerns are not with any particular educational institution or arrangement. He is setting out the methodology of a new form of education. In Rousseau's work, we see that education has a social aim. This is to produce the citizen who will voluntarily act in accordance with the civil or 'general will'. They will do this in the same way that individuals in a state of nature act in their own self-interest (Perkinson 1980: 145). Pupils or students must learn from nature or things. The teacher must facilitate learning so that pupils or students learn for themselves.

Task 1.13: Learning from nature

Is learning best undertaken by learning for oneself? How far is your own practice governed by concepts that might be compatible with Rousseau's idea of not interfering directly in the educational process for fear of corrupting learning?

Further reading: the clearest statement of Rousseau's philosophy is given in the Books I–III of *Émile*. Book V which covers the 'last act in the drama of youth' might be of more interest to the teacher in PCE.

Dewey

John Dewey (1859–1952): Professor of Philosophy at the University of Chicago from 1894. Major educational works: *Democracy and Education* (1916) and *Experience and Education* (1938).

'If in our own time the distinction between education in the traditional sense and vocational training, as increasingly demanded by a technological society, has become somewhat blurred, this is in part due to the influence of Dewey's work' (Russell [1959] 1989: 296). In the four decades since Russell asserted this balanced judgement, Dewey's work is still a subject for fierce criticism and passionate praise. For example, journalist Melanie Phillips has recently criticized Dewey's emphasis on process over product (knowledge) and argued that his influence on education has been 'malign, revolutionary and destructive' (Phillips 1996: 210). While Professor Frank Coffield claims that Phillips has misunderstood Dewey and agrees with him that education is the 'fundamental method of social progress' and is about 'the formation of proper social life' (Coffield 1997).

Dewey's writings encourage such different interpretations. They are written with a radical reforming zeal that often masks the kernel of what he is saying. For teachers in PCE the key element of interest in Dewey's work is his concern with vocational education and with using this to make education more relevant to students. It is important to understand what Dewey actually said because he is the most influential and frequently quoted philosopher in the PCE field, and because his work is subject to various interpretations. (It would also be useful before tackling the discussion of vocationalism in Section 1.4 below.)

In *Democracy and Education* (1916) Dewey warns against the separation in modern society between the capacities of the young and the concerns of the adult. Direct sharing in the pursuits of adults becomes increasingly difficult. Therefore teaching in formal institutions becomes necessary. This teaching is less personal and vital, and formal instruction 'easily becomes remote and dead – abstract and bookish' (Dewey [1916] 1966: 8).

The teaching of subjects is held to be 'specialist' teaching. The 'technical philosopher' could be 'ill advised in his actions and judgement outside of his speciality': 'Isolation of subject matter from a social context is the chief obstruction in current practice to securing a general training of mind. Literature, art, religion, when thus disassociated, are just as narrowing as the technical things which the professional upholders of general education strenuously oppose' (Dewey [1916] 1966: 67). One of the ways of overcoming this is to ensure that the child's native experience is not undervalued and that 'active occupations' form the basis of all teaching. This is the nearest Dewey comes to being 'child-centred'. What his injunction intends is obviously achieved by the introduction of subjects such as gardening, woodwork and cooking, but for mathematics and science: 'Even for older students the social sciences would be less abstract and formal if they were dealt with less as sciences (less as formulated bodies of knowledge) and more in their direct subject-matter as that is found in the daily life of the social groups in which the student shares' (Dewey [1916] 1966: 201).

Dewey criticizes the individualism of Rousseau and sees 'natural development' as an aim of education, but one only partially stated if it refers only to our primitive powers. He sees nurture not as corrupting but as

the development of those natural powers ([1916] 1966: 111–18, 123). There is, however, a particularly American form of individualism in Dewey, who accepted the myth of the frontier as something that had elevated American society from the worst features of the development of European capitalism. In this sense, he looks back to a pre-industrial world in which there is a harmony between learning and adult life. This leaves him closer to Rousseau than he thinks. The difference is that he believes that industrialization has created the possibility for a truly democratic society which can be achieved through education.

Ryan is correct to point out, in opposition to Dewey's cruder critics, that he was *not* arguing that 'the point of industrial training was to produce a docile workforce adapted to the needs of capitalist employers' (Ryan 1995: 177). Dewey thought that capitalism was at best a semiambulant corpse but rejected the revolutionary route (Ryan 1995: 178). The central chapter in Dewey's book is Chapter 7, 'The Democratic Conception in Education' (Dewey [1916] 1966: 81–99). He sets out a vision for education in terms of an end to the separation into classes by ending the division between 'mental' and 'manual' labour. This is experienced as the division between those who receive a 'liberal education' and those that receive something poorer, or mere training for work. He envisages an education that reflects the democratic ideal. Democracy is a form of associated living, with numerous and varied points of contact with a plurality of social groups which in itself will perpetuate democracy (Dewey [1916] 1966: 86–8). Education shares these ideals and is therefore essential to democratic society.

Some writers have held Dewey's chapter on vocationalism to be the poorest in the book. It is, however, Dewey's clearest attempt to spell out the implications of his earlier chapters. Dewey defines vocationalism as 'such a direction of life activities as renders them perceptibly significant to a person because of the consequences they accomplish, and also useful to his associates' (Dewey [1916] 1966: 307) It is neither 'narrowly practical' nor 'merely pecuniary'. A later summary adds a temporal requirement: 'A vocation is any form of continuous activity which renders service to others and engages personal powers on behalf of the accomplishment of results' (Dewey [1916] 1966: 319). There is a clear emphasis here on the utility of what is undertaken to 'others' or society. The definition is also so general it covers activities we would not normally call vocational. For example it includes academic study and scholarship as a vocation, as training for an academic 'career'. But here the question of 'utility', especially to society, makes no sense and can only be destructive of the quest for knowledge by subjecting it to the requirement of producing results or being useful to society (Anderson 1980b: 139–40).

Dewey claims that 'the only adequate training *for* occupations is in training *through* occupations' (Dewey [1916] 1966: 310, emphasis as original). He argues that industrial society has created the necessity and possibility for educational reorganization but 'there is a danger that vocational education will be interpreted in theory and practice as trade education' ([1916] 1966: 316). The only way of avoiding this is the methodological

one of producing in the schools 'a projection of the type of society we should like to realise, and by forming minds in accord with it gradually modify the larger and more recalcitrant features of adult society' ([1916] 1966: 317).

Dewey sees education as essential to the achievement of a democratic society. By reflecting that society in its organization, it will ensure that democracy comes into being or continues to develop and change. He stresses the importance of the pupil's or student's *experience* and of socially relevant activities or '*occupations*' in the classroom. Dewey recognizes the dangers in how people may take his suggestions and rejects narrow training for work as a definition of 'vocational education'.

Task 1.14: Dewey: for or against?

Dewey sets education the project of building a democratic society. How far are you in sympathy with this aim? Consider how it differs from the aim of education for Socrates and Rousseau.

These three philosophies of education will appear in discussions of curriculum ideology in broad categories such as classical humanism, humanism and social reconstructionism (Chapter 7) and in learning theory (Chapter 3) when cognitive, humanistic and empirical theories are discussed (behaviourism is merely an example of the latter). When working through these discussions, relate them to the philosophical positions outlined here. Remember that they may not always be distinct.

The 'triumph' of vocationalism

KEY ISSUES

'Vocational education' is understood in a variety of ways

According to one particular view, questions of value and value judgement are outside its sphere

Many have sought to reconcile vocational and liberal education

The essential elements of the new educational initiatives of the 1980s could be said to fit a special needs deficit model

The potential of technology to transform lives is the subject of a wide range of views from those of a variety of political persuasions

Task 1.15

Try to describe what you understand by 'vocational education'. Review your statement when you have finished reading this section.

The aim of this section is to examine how 'vocationalism' has come to dominate thinking across the whole of PCE. It is related to the general themes we have discussed in the two previous sections: the attack upon 'academic' or subject-based knowledge and Dewey's criticism of the arid and dry nature of formal education. It is our contention that vocationalism has triumphed in the sense that it dominates our thinking and that Tony Blair's three priorities for Britain 'education, education, education' could refer to an impoverished notion of education dominated by vocationalism.

Vocationalism is a term used to refer to various theories, ideological positions and some simplistic attitudes that have attempted to link the world of work to a greater or lesser degree with education. Such approaches often suggest that, as work is an important part of life, we should find a place for it in schools and colleges (Lewis 1997). But the variety of these theories and the unanalysed popular usage of terms can seem confusing or, worse still, simply unproblematic. The situation is so chronic that one set of academics has been led to declare that: 'No single characteristic defines this new vocationalism. It is marked by variety of policies and programmes and diversity of action and actors. But it is guided, if not propelled, by a determination to establish closer and better interrelationships between the experience of both formative education and preparatory training and the working world' (Skilbeck *et al.* 1994: 2).

A general trend we can identify at the outset is for vocationalist initiatives to be presented as part of a package of a supposedly radical rethinking of the aims of education, or providing the basis for reforms leading to a more relevant or modern, technologically-based education. They often claim to be more democratic, offering a better education for the masses rather than a pale shadow of the elitist education offered to the better-off or to specific social groups. The terminology of the theorists of vocationalism can be particularly confusing. For example, we come across one theorist arguing for a 'critical vocationalism' (Donald 1992). Intellectual acrobatics are required even to attempt to understand what this could possibly mean. On a more everyday level, we find teachers using the phrase 'vocational education' in relation to a variety of courses, which may have some educational element, or may simply be training courses. Either way, there is no doubt that the advocates of the priority of practice over knowledge have triumphed. Frequent references to the 'vocational element in education' are seen as unremarkable. It is, however, possible to argue for an education that is entirely theoretical and to see it as a duty to combat those who would promote an education that is in any way practical. This would be the traditional position of the liberal educator.

However extreme this view may seem, it is coherent and deserves attention (Anderson 1980c: 157).

There does seem to be a consistent refusal by participants in debates about vocationalism to recognize important conceptual distinctions. The Kennedy Report, *Learning Works* (Kennedy 1997b), talks throughout in an undiscriminating way about 'learning'. Kennedy makes no attempt to analyse what we mean by 'learning' in different contexts. Thus learning to use a lathe, to chop vegetables, learning citizenship, mathematics and ancient languages are given a spurious equality. The treatment of complex philosophical distinctions and debates as easily resolved or as semantic questions reaches its apogee in the introduction to the third Dearing Report (Dearing 1997). Here we find Dearing declaring with unmasked enthusiasm that the near future will see the *'historic boundaries between vocational and academic education breaking down*, with increasingly active partnerships between higher education institutions and the worlds of industry, commerce and public service' (p. 8, our emphasis). Dearing writes as if the 'academic' and 'vocational' divide was something totally unproblematic to be resolved through the mutual respect of the partners as they work together.

The recognition of an academic and vocational divide has been part of the debate about the nature of education for over 2000 years. Aristotle in the *Politics* notes that in his own day 'nobody knows' whether the young should be trained in studies that are useful 'as a means of livelihood' or to 'promote virtue' or in the 'higher studies' (discussed in Lester Smith 1957: 11). The point is not that nothing changes; this would be ahistorical, as ancient Greek society and Britain today bear no comparison. But at least it is apparent from Aristotle that the Greeks felt that there was a real and important problem here. Contemporary discussions are simply trivial and sanguine by comparison.

It is the intention in this section to provide an introduction to what should be a real debate by providing a critical guide to the discussions of the various types of vocationalism that have manifested themselves since James Callaghan (the Labour prime minister 1976–79) launched the 'Great Debate'. We deliberately restrict our use of the label 'new' vocationalism because, if it has any meaning, it applies only to one very particular post-war period.

The way we think now

To understand the sense in which vocationalism is triumphant, it is worthwhile locating it within a more general intellectual malaise. This has been well described by writer and critic Richard Hoggart, who sees contemporary Britain as being swamped by a tidal wave of relativism, which he defines as 'the obsessive avoidance of judgements of quality or moral judgement' (Hoggart 1996: 3). One element of this dominant mood is the acceptance of vocationalism at all levels of the educational system. Arguments about improving the quality of life, or turning around Britain's economic performance, are often supported by talk of the need for skills

training, or of the promotion of some form of vocational education or training. This is apparently a 'classless impulse' (Hoggart 1996: 220), but, Hoggart argues, only to those who oppose the traditional notion of education being a good in itself, whatever its practical benefits. It does seem to be true that vocationalism, as a standpoint which avoids debate and discussion about important differences of value, is widespread. A glimpse of the extent of the obsession with the vocational is apparent from the following passage from *The Economist* (1996):

> On the face of it, the case for generous public support for training is strong. Unskilled people are much more likely to be out of work than skilled ones; if only their qualifications could be improved, they might find jobs more readily. Not only would they benefit, but so would the economy as a whole. A better-trained productive workforce would be a more productive one; so more training ought to mean not just lower unemployment but faster growth and higher living standards. Unions like training programmes because they can use them to push up wages. Academics like them because they increase demand for education. Parents like them because they give out-of-work, out-of-school youths something to do. Prophets of a post-modern society praise them as part of an ethic of lifelong learning. And employers don't mind because the public pays the bill.

Everyone is in favour of training. A recent study showed that a massive 66 per cent of workers thought that education and training were *the* means of progressing their careers (Hudson *et al.* 1996). There is constant discussion in the media about a 'skills gap' (IRDAC 1990) to be filled by training. But *The Economist* simply refers to training for work rather than vocational education. This is sometimes referred to as 'vocationalism' in its old or traditional sense of training to do a job. The argument of the article is that the most successful training takes place in the workplace and is provided by employers, as opposed to training provided by the state or its quangos. This may be true but it is dynamic economies which are referred to to illustrate the argument. There is a chicken and egg question to be resolved here. Is the problem identified as a 'skills gap' a result of relative economic decline or its cause? Any skills gap which does exist must surely be resolved at the political or economic level and not by scapegoating the employed and unemployed as unskilled. It could, indeed, be seen as a 'jobs gap'. In fact the debate about a 'skills gap' is one-sided, being largely promoted by employers' organizations. When asked to specify skills needed, most employers provide answers in terms of moral or personal qualities that have little to do with 'skills' in the sense that most people understand the term. We think of a skill in a traditional way as relating to, say, carpentry, engineering or IT. However, the skills needed at work are usually those that can be learned in a few weeks with minimal difficulty. The dynamic of industry is to reduce, diminish or replace such skills (Marx [1867] 1974: 407–8, 457–8; Korndörffer 1991: 222–3). Even in the case of IT, it is far from certain that we are at the dawn of a 'new era' or 'knowledge age' (Woudhuysen 1997). It is important to recognize that there is a debate here that is closely related to our assumptions about whether we face a 'skills gap' or 'job gap'.

Task 1.16

Looking at your own area of expertise, identify any 'skills' that are in short supply. Are the skills you identified technical, educational or personal? Could they be met within PCE?

Liberal education (early twentieth century)

There have been many attempts to analyse various forms of vocationalism, and most of these attempt to reconcile 'vocational' and 'liberal' education (e.g. Williams 1994: 97–8). In Britain, the traditional or 'narrow view' of vocationalism as 'training for a job' was mostly rejected by educational reformers. R. H. Tawney was perhaps the best-known writer whom we associate with this line of thinking (Tawney 1922). Not only conservatives or traditionalists but also most socialists and radicals sought a decent liberal education in traditional and modern subjects for everyone. Access to the whole of humanity's cultural inheritance was the demand that was made. What was good enough for the sons of the masters was good enough for the workers. Vocational training was held to be entirely a matter for employers. This does not mean that individuals did not seek vocational training, but the traditional position was against vocationalism. This must be stressed as it is now almost forgotten, particularly by proponents of a 'democratic' education. According to this view, there is simply no connection between 'education' and 'training'. It could be argued that work-related training does go on in schools and colleges, but this does not establish anything other than an organizational connection between the two.

Training for jobs (the 1960s)

In the 1960s, employers relied upon the state to provide training in technical colleges but the employer was responsible for the day release of young employees. The lack of system in this method of training led to its being called 'stop gap' or 'gap filling' by many critics (Hall 1994: 43–5), but whatever its faults, it was clearly related to training for jobs. When Harold Wilson spoke to the 1962 Labour Party conference of forging a new Britain in the 'white heat of the technological revolution' there was no other conception in anyone's mind but real training for real jobs. The main debates were about 'upskilling' the workforce. This is a reminder that talk of technological revolution is not new and in the 1960s the technological revolution put man on the moon (compare Ainley 1988: 143

who argues 'technological change is developing exponentially'). We can consider vocationalism as training for jobs as the major form of training up to the mid-1970s.

Training without jobs (the 1970s)

In the 1970s, economic crisis and rising youth unemployment changed things. One clear consequence of James Callaghan's 'Great Debate' was the systematic involvement of industry in the planning of the educational process. There were other elements too. The increasing role of the state in directing vocational training in a time of financial cutback has been well discussed (Benn and Fairley 1986; Finn 1987; Ainley 1988, 1990). The training on offer was still largely related to jobs. It is important to remember the general antagonism and resistance there was to the various adult and youth training initiatives. There were youth protests and opposition from the trade unions, trades councils and political groups. The main criticisms were of 'slave labour' schemes or the use of 'cheap labour' to replace existing jobs. Out of this grew an emphasis on pre-vocational and basic skills training. This transitional period is one in which the concept of 'vocationalism' starts to shift in meaning from 'day release' or 'stop gap' provision towards 'pre-vocational provision'. We could date it as beginning in 1976 but its fullest flowering is in the period of the Youth Training Scheme (YTS) from 1983 to1989. Most analyses focus on the increasing or changed form of state involvement with the training of young people (see Hickox 1995). While these discussions are important it is our argument that the curriculum developments proposed help us understand the long-term impact of these changes rather than simply seeing them as a matter of the state crudely forcing young people into years of slave labour.

The 'new' vocationalism (the 1980s)

Employers in this crisis situation were asking: why should we be training young workers who cannot benefit from work because of their attitudes, lack of basic skills or poor discipline? Although this attitude ran counter to the facts, it became the basis of the Manpower Services Commission's (MSC) development of a range of training initiatives, culminating in the YTS, which were available to all unemployed young people. This pre-vocationalism is the basis of what came to be called the 'new' vocationalism. What was on offer was a curriculum derived from special needs programmes based on the sort of personal and social training necessary to prepare youngsters with learning difficulties for the world of work. The limitations of these pre-vocational courses and initiatives did not stop them being successful as a stage in the development of vocationalism.

YTS can be seen as a failure if judged by comparison with earlier vocational training in the narrow sense, and as a pre-vocational scheme. It provided employment for only two-thirds of the trainees who completed the courses and this employment was often short term. The only vocational element in these courses was an increasingly tenuous belief on the part of the providers that young people could get a job. However, there were wider forces influencing young people and their teachers. This was the decade in which the Further Education Unit (FEU) produced its influential documents winning over the newer college lecturer with curriculum-based papers. Lower-level technical college courses and private training courses sprang up all over the country funded by the MSC. The Technical and Vocational Education Initiative (TVEI) gave educational developments and experiment a free rein. The labour market reality of the time was that there was no work in the traditional sense of a job for life. Employment was going to be intermittent and temporary, and life at college was better than unemployment. A traditional life pattern of the time was for young people to move from a YTS to employment, then on to a college course or evening class, then into a period of unemployment and than back into another, adult, training scheme. Many of those who worked in colleges or were real or potential trainees were totally sceptical about the value of these courses. But a lumpen scepticism is entirely passive: the pragmatic lessons of unemployment had been learned, and youth rebellion did not materialize. The unions and the Trades Union Congress (TUC) came back on-side to discuss training. A credit-led boom brought the yuppie into temporary being, and in this climate there was the expectation that you could make it and find a job but you were on your own.

The new vocationalism is often seen as a Thatcherite victory in creating an employer-dominated training scheme for young people. The early opposition to Youth Opportunities Programme (YOP) and YTS faded away leaving only a few radical educationalists arguing for something better. However, many of those opposing YTS schemes did not see them as a betrayal of the ideal of a liberal education for all, but the failure to provide something different. These writers were influenced by Marx and Engels' occasional comments on education (Marx [1867] 1974: 453–4, [1875] 1968: 329; Engels [1878] 1975: 378–82) and generally promote technological education. For example, Willis (1987) and Ainley (1990, 1993) argue that the working classes need to improve their skills for sale on the market and radical thinkers do them a disservice by not arguing for a form of vocational education that will meet their needs as a class. Willis (1987: xvii) puts this case well: 'how is it, and is it, possible to reconcile the tensions between training as class reproduction and training as working-class interest more in the favour of the working class?' Ainley (1993: 93) sees technological advance as the answer: 'In a modernising economy, education and training must raise the skills of all workers from the bottom up . . . Education and training will then integrate rather than separate mental and manual labour . . . New technology provides the potential to enable all working people to become multiskilled and flexible in a true sense . . .'. Precursors of these views include Harold Wilson's populist technological revolution in the 1960s and the 'post-Fordist' utopian visions of the 1980s. Such arguments have been savagely attacked as being unrelated to the reality of contemporary capitalism (Roberts *et al.* 1994), as this level of training would simply make employment too expensive. With an eye on profits there is no possibility that employers or the state would promote such training and the result would be redundancy for the mass of workers who would be too expensive to employ (*see* Yaffe 1978: 12–13). The illusion lies in a belief in the power of technology to transform people's lives rather than a political movement doing so, which has been a popular view since the end of the cold war. But such views are not necessarily implied by a Marxist analysis as Brian Simon proved in his defence of liberal education in response to the 'Great Debate' (Simon 1985). The consequence of arguments about the possibility of a new industrial revolution which will benefit workers is a convergence of the views of the 'left' and of the 'right', represented by employers. There is therefore no real opposition to vocationalism, only opposition to its crudest forms.

Education without jobs (the 1990s)

The period from 1989 to the present can be seen as one of containment. The number of young people staying on in FE increased dramatically to 89 per cent of all 16-year-olds, and led Nick Tate, the head of the School Curriculum and Assessment Authority (SCAA), to comment in the summer of 1997 that the effective school leaving age was now 18. With 30 per cent of all young people going on to HE and many into other training schemes, we might make the effective leaving age 21 or even higher. The mass expansion of FE and HE has few critics, and even they see some basis to be positive about aspects of the work of the new universities (Ainley 1994). This period of containment is also the period of the qualification explosion. Demand for NVQs, GNVQs, GCSEs, A levels, degrees, credit bearing courses and in-service qualifications seems never ending. The expansion of qualifications available and the apparent improvement in their attainment by young people has been questioned, and one writer is notorious for calling the whole thing a sham (Phillips 1996). Certainly, qualifications are now required for jobs that were previously thought to be unskilled, such as classroom assistants. We need to ask if there is any element of vocationalism here. Perhaps only in the residual sense of 'employability' which was a theme that grew out of government papers and reports in the mid-1990s (DfEE 1995a) and is highlighted in the Report of the Commission on Social Justice (CSJ 1994: 175–6). Employability is divorced from vocational skills or even from pre-vocational skills, so why even refer to 'employability' as having to do with jobs at all? Why not just talk of 'learning' and 'education'? This is certainly a popular move with politicians, and educationalists are also seeking a move away from vocationalism: 'Serious attention now needs to be given to educating as opposed to training a majority of the population hitherto denied access to further and higher education' (Avis *et al.* 1996: 180).

So, is vocationalism defeated? The answer is 'no'. Mainstream education is dominated by the vocational themes of a work-related, often competence-based curriculum, the introduction of pre-vocational or personal and social development under the guise of 'employability' and above all, by the supposed need to adapt to a life in a new 'communication' or 'technological' age. Education as a whole has become vocationalized in the sense that the connection between the world of work and education is seen as necessary rather than contingent. What this means is that, whereas people once thought that the knowledge gained in getting an education was not irrelevant to the workplace, now the sort of knowledge that is on offer seems to be only that that *is* relevant to work. Even to lecturers in vocational areas, this must be seen as a complete debasement of knowledge. As mentioned above, the Dearing Report (Dearing 1997) sets out exactly this model for the development of HE. Even if we call for a return to 'educating' rather than 'training', what is likely to be provided is not a liberal education but a poor vocationalized replacement. The same can be said of the Kennedy Report (Kennedy 1997b) with its promotion of life-long learning. What is being offered is an 'education' that amounts to learning up to NVQ Level 3 – a *vocational* standard, and one that it set very low. This has parallels with the 'back to basics' drives promoted by some ministers that make Britain sound like a Third World country. Standards are being set but set much lower than they were at the time of the Robbins Report (Robbins 1963). Vocationalism is triumphant but it appears disguised as education. Perhaps the main challenge for PCE teachers in the new millennium is showing that the emperor has no clothes.

Task 1.17

We have looked at vocationalism in several forms, as narrow training, as pre-vocational training, as being concerned with employability, and in a 'back to basics' or 'educational' manifestation. These have been identified with particular historical periods. What would you envisage as a model of PCE for the new millennium?

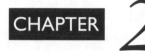

CHAPTER 2

THE POST-COMPULSORY TEACHER: LEARNING AND DEVELOPING

2.1 What is Chapter 2 about?

This book assumes that its readers will be engaged in a programme of training or staff development and be teaching or on teaching practice. This chapter will therefore consider ways in which teachers and trainers will learn and how such learning processes can focus on their professional context. In addition, our experience has been that many students, although knowledgeable and expert in their own trade, profession or curriculum area, have not been involved in systematic study, sometimes for many years, and this chapter will therefore act as an introduction to the skills required for using such learning, supporting the transition from subject experts to managers of others' learning.

Section 2.2 considers different notions of 'the good teacher'. You should be clear about what you understand by this as a basis for your own development as well as examining how your professional context may help or hinder this development. Section 2.3 considers techniques of self-evaluation, while Section 2.4 looks at the value of classroom observation, of and by you. Section 2.5 addresses the potential of using peers as a learning resource before Section 2.6 looks at the process of planning and researching a written assignment.

2.2 *Teacher learning and development*

KEY ISSUES

Effective teacher development assumes a model of 'the good teacher'

Notions of the good teacher vary in what features they emphasize

Professional development cannot take place unless learning is applied to the teacher's own professional context

Our ideas about how teachers can effectively learn and develop must be connected with our notion of what makes a good teacher.

Task 2.1: Our own experience

2.1(a) Consider your experiences as a learner when at school and since then. What qualities did good teachers have? What qualities did bad teachers lack?

2.1(b) Share these views with the rest of the group.

Figure 2.1 shows the responses of a group of AE teachers to Task 2.1. Responses such as those shown in Figure 2.1 tend to focus on three aspects of teaching, and these are defined in Figure 2.2. You may notice that the three aspects broadly correspond with Bloom's (1964) classification of educational objectives into cognitive, psycho-motor and affective domains. The kind of learning which we feel will make someone a better teacher will depend upon the value we place on each aspect. Nationally, policy has swung between all three aspects. In the 1960s there was a move away from 'teacher training' to 'teacher education', a desire to emphasize the knowledge-based academic content of the then new BEd degree in contrast to previous skill-oriented programmes. But in the last ten years, teacher education, along with training across many vocational areas, has moved towards learning in the second and third aspects, which can be broadly termed a 'competency-based approach'.

Task 2.2: Your own priorities

2.2(a) Looking at the three aspects in Figure 2.1, which aspects of teaching do you feel you need to focus on to make you a better teacher?

2.2(b) Share your thoughts with the group. Where the emphasis differs, how do you account for this? Contrasting subjects taught? Differing institutions? Variety in personal and professional background and experience?

Figure 2.1 AE teachers' responses to Task 2.1

'I remember getting interested in history for the first time when I did an evening course. The tutor had a passion for it.'

'He was clearly a brilliant physicist but he couldn't get his ideas over.'

'However frustrated you became, this teacher had limitless patience.'

'She seemed to be able to help you because she'd experienced the same difficulties herself.'

'We never learned anything because we didn't listen to him. And we didn't listen to him because we didn't respect him.'

'She seemed to make learning even the most routine things fun.'

'He had the ability to bring the subject to life.'

'He couldn't control our class. We soon found he couldn't control any class.'

'She could always explain even the most difficult things in terms you could understand.'

'He didn't seem to enjoy being with students.'

Figure 2.2 Three key aspects of teaching

Subject knowledge and expertise
Those thought of as good teachers tend to know their subjects, either through study or experience or both. But this is no guarantee of effectiveness: a very common experience is of the knowledgeable teacher who can't communicate.

Skills and abilities
Whether controlling a class, communicating or understanding learning difficulties, the good teacher is seen as one who demonstrates skills and abilities to a high degree.

Commitment and emotions
This third aspect is wide-ranging but includes references to 'enthusiasm', 'passion', 'caring' and 'patience' – all qualities to do with emotions, attitudes and dispositions.

You should now have a clearer notion of your own learning priorities. But, unless that learning is effectively applied to your practice, unless it makes a difference to your teaching, professional development is unlikely to take place. Sections 2.3, 2.4, and 2.5 will look in detail at the ways in

Figure 2.3 Contexts in which teaching takes place

Your institution
Is it a large college, a small adult centre, the training section of a public service or industrial/commercial organization? How do you fit into it? What resources and support are available to you?

The extent to which you work with others
Do you work closely with colleagues as part of a course team for example, or do you attend an evening centre once a week, meeting only your students? Do you have a line manager? If not, to whom are you accountable?

Degree of professional autonomy
Who decides what you teach? Is there a detailed syllabus? Can you determine content and sequence?

Student targeting and recruitment
Do you control this or does the institution?

which you might reflect on your practice, but consider for a moment the current context in which you teach. It will have a number of important features, shown in Figure 2.3.

Task 2.3: Your professional context

2.3(a) Describe your own professional context in the light of the features above.

2.3(b) Given your context, what aspects of it might help or hinder your professional development? Share this with the group. How might common barriers to development be overcome?

 ## *Self-evaluation*

KEY ISSUES

Self-evaluation, narrowly or widely focused, requires you to assess how far aims and obejctives have been realized in students' learning experience

Self-review of lessons can be distorted by subjectivity

There are techniques such as videotaping and student questionnaires which can supplement self-review with more objective data

Perhaps the major tool which will lead to your development as a teacher is self-evaluation. The nature of this evaluation will depend on the focus you give it. It could have a wide focus where you consider several or all aspects of the learning session involved, or a more narrow focus, such as the evaluation focusing on learning needs shown in Example 2.1 on page 32. Other objects of a narrow-focus evaluation might be:

- planning and preparation;
- teaching and learning strategies;
- communication skills and techniques;
- group management;
- managing a variety of student behavioural characteristics;
- learning resources;
- management of the learning environment;
- assessment.

Task 2.4: Choosing a focus for self-evaluation

2.4(a) Select a lesson you have recently taught. Jot down the main points for evaluation using a narrow-focus topic chosen from the list above.

2.4(b) Do certain lessons rather than others suggest themselves for a narrowly-focused evaluation?

However widely or narrowly focused, your evaluation should attempt to measure how far your aims and objectives have been met. Of course, you may have realized as the lesson progressed that particular aim(s) and objective(s) were paramount and you wished to concentrate on related activities, or that unplanned learning, a frequent and often very pleasing outcome of a learning session, had taken place. However, overall, the process of evaluation is an estimation of how far the aims and objectives have been met in terms of student learning.

Task 2.5: Self-evaluation

Look at the lesson plan and self-evaluation in Example 2.1. How successful is the teacher in her or his evaluation at considering the lesson's effectiveness in realizing the aims and objectives specified?

Example 2.1

LESSON PLAN

Venue: North Kent College *Course:* Vocational Access
Room: F16   *Group:* 1st Year

Example 2.1 (Cont'd)

Date: 22.1.98.   *No. of students:* 15

Time: 10am–11am   *Subject:* Communications

                                              Topic: Introduction to self-presentation

Aims:

- To introduce students to what influences and determines judgements we make about each other.
- To help students understand the dangers of making superficial judgements about others
- To bring about an awareness of how students are seen by others in a variety of situations

Objectives: At the end of the session, students will be able to:

- describe how far they under- or overestimate qualities in themselves;
- specify examples of when they have misread others' reactions;
- understand the consequences of gender and cultural stereotyping;
- imagine the effects of their self-presentation on others in a variety of situations.

	Content	*Teacher activities*	*Student activities*	*Resources*
10:00–10:20	Self-image	• Instructions on how to complete table • Support of pair work • Lead group discussion	• Complete table • Work with partner • Group discussion	Blank attitude questionnaires
10:20–10:40	First impressions/ stereotyping	• Set task • One-to-one support • Lead group discussion	• Describe features of people in photographs • Group discussion	Sets of photographs
10:40–11:00	Effect of own self-presentation in a variety of situations	• One-to one support • Lead plenary discussion	• Write down descriptions of how perceived • Take part in plenary discussion	

Example 2.1 (Cont'd)

EVALUATION

Focus: Learning needs

A consideration of self-presentation and an awareness of how others see us is particularly important at this stage of the course: none of these youngsters has been, for any length of time, in a workplace and they're soon going to be meeting a range of adults they probably haven't encountered before when they go out on their first work experience in two weeks' time. Anxiety about how they'll cope with this on a personal level came up frequently in the needs analysis. In addition, an alarming degree of prejudice emerged in the group during early discussions and I want to introduce stereotyping as an issue as part of the course, as something they should take on board as an aspect of their relationships and communication with others.

It's clear that few of the group have thought hard about themselves and a resistance to this was, I think, at the heart of A and G's disruptive behaviour during the session. A second factor could have been to do with their perception of talk, of discussion as not 'real' work: it was noticeable that the only point at which they applied themselves during the session was in the final task when there was writing involved.

The second task on photographs went better than the first: I realized how much easier it was for the students to grasp ideas presented and dealt with visually than in an abstract form in a table. Also, the students seemed to enjoy imagining who these people were – the most creative aspect of the session.

Overall, from the point of view of learning needs, I felt the students, though generally interested, needed to be more active and I intend to use role-play in the next session. I also intend to use more visual stimuli. Finally, I think I was too ambitious with this group, expecting them to grasp too many complex concepts in the time available and I shall look carefully at the content of the next session in this respect.

You may have thought this teacher to have been only partially successful in judging how far his or her aims and objectives were achieved in the session taught. This is, to some extent, because we are often far more certain about student learning problems and difficulties than about whether we know what they have learnt. But part of the difficulty of making evaluative judgements about students' experiences in our classrooms is how subjective these are and how problematic it can be both to teach and observe a group at the same time. The first of two possibly more objective strategies is considered in Figure 2.4.

Figure 2.4 Strategy 1: videotaping

The following entry was made in the teacher's reflective log for the Vocational Access group session on 22.1.98:

'What struck me most dramatically when I played the video back were physical and vocal aspects of my performance that I'd never been aware of before: my voice does tend to be monotonous – it needs to be far more expressive; and I have a habit, which must be irritating, of moving my arms about in a way which bears no relation to what I'm talking about! I noticed in supporting the pair work that I wasn't keeping an eye on how the other pairs were doing, whether they were in difficulty and wanted my attention. When I did move on, it tended to be to the pair who were most vociferous. My management of group discussion was reasonable but I did notice how I was rather impatient in question and answer if the answer wasn't forthcoming quickly enough. When explaining points, I just didn't persevere enough with alternative explanations when individual students were still unclear, since I was anxious about covering all the ground in the time available.'

Task 2.6: Comparing strategies

Compare the analysis in Figure 2.4 with the teacher's self-evaluation in Example 2.1. Which *specific* points in the video recording might have been difficult for the teacher to have been aware of from her or his own observation?

The second strategy is the student questionnaire. On the face of it, it seems odd to distribute a questionnaire to students you see on a regular basis, but a questionnaire is a more objective evaluation technique than others and has the following main advantages:

- students are more likely to be open and honest than when directly questioned;
- the questions can elicit more specific responses;
- individual anonymous completion reduces the possibility of conformity of response.

The major drawback is that it is not as easy as it appears to construct even the most simple questionnaire, one difficulty being composing questions of the appropriate type and wording to produce clear, useful information.

Judith Bell, in her excellent *Doing Your Research Project* (1987), refers to Youngman's (1986) question types, in particular:

- *Verbal or open:* The answer expected is a word, phrase or comment, which can make these responses difficult to analyse, e.g. 'What did you feel about the discussion session?'

- *List:* A list of items is offered for the respondent to choose from, e.g. 'Tick any of the following if it describes your motivation for coming on this course':

  1 To improve my prospects of getting a job
  2 Out of interest
  3 To keep up with my children's schoolwork
  4 I need the skills involved at work

- *Category:* Respondents classify themselves as falling into one of a number of categories, e.g. 'State whether you are':

  1 Employed full-time
  2 Employed part-time
  3 Self-employed
  4 Unemployed

- *Ranking:* A series of qualities is given to be put into a rank order, e.g. 'Place the following in their order of importance to you: pleasant classroom environment; good catering facilities; accessible library; wide range of learning resources.'

- *Scale:* Various kinds of scale or continuum give students the opportunity to choose the appropriate point on the scale as in the example below.

	Strongly agree	*Agree*	*Neither agree or disagree*	*Disagree*	*Strongly disagree*
1 Academic support was effective					
2 Tutors marked and returned work promptly					
3 Accommodation was suitable					
4 Teaching was of high quality					

Bell (1987) also draws attention to the potential dangers inherent in question wording, and these are shown in Figure 2.5.

Figure 2.5 Dangers inherent in question wording

Ambiguity, imprecision, assumption	Could your question mean different things to different students (e.g. 'Would you describe yourself as able, average or not very good?'), be unclear about the kind of answer required, or already contain an answer within it?
Memory	Does the question rely too heavily on students' memories, which may be unreliable? (e.g. 'What level of basic skills did you achieve at school?').
Knowledge	Does the question presuppose the possession of information the students don't have? (e.g. 'Who sets the fee levels in your local education authority?').
Double questions	Are there two questions present in one? (e.g. 'Did you feel the role play and interview were worthwhile?').
Leading questions	Does the question lead you to a particular response? (e.g. 'Don't you think communication is the most important part of your job?').
Hypothetical questions	'If you could change this lesson, how would you do it?' A pointless question, if it is clear to the students they won't have that power.

Source: Bell 1987: 60–4.

Task 2.7: Devising a questionnaire

2.7(a) Devise a short questionnaire focusing on a lesson or series of lessons.

2.7(b) Exchange this with a partner's and comment on question type and wording. Discuss common problems with the group.

2.7(c) Administer the questionnaire to the relevant students.

2.7(d) Analyse the results, question by question.

2.7(e) Once you've analysed the results, summarize them for the rest of your group. Consider how useful the information is to you. Does any of it confirm or conflict with that gained through other evaluation methods? How might you change practice as a result of this exercise?

Observation

> KEY ISSUES
>
> Observation offers a more objective evaluation technique than self-evaluation
>
> It is important for both observer and observed to be clear about their roles and the purpose of the observation
>
> Most observation will use a qualitative rather than a quantitative approach, creating the potential for problems of interpretation

Traditionally, teachers have enjoyed a degree of professional autonomy, and there is still a strong proprietorial feeling among many about teaching their own students in their own classroom. So, however experienced and professionally confident teachers are, being observed by others, whether they be colleagues, line managers or supervising tutors, is often a stressful experience. Paradoxically, however, such observation of and by others can be the basis of some of the most useful professional reflection we can undertake. As with evaluation strategies like the videotaping and questionnaire considered in Section 2.3, feedback from observation offers a more objective viewpoint on your work (although this can be complicated by questions of interpretation, dealt with below). The difference here is that the feedback is 'live', given immediately in an interactive context.

Many teachers do have reservations about being observed: the presence of a stranger in their classroom is bound to affect both their students and themselves, they argue, making the observed session unnatural and artificial and therefore reducing the value of the feedback given. There are many factors, of course, which will affect how both teachers and students behave when a visitor is present: how used they are to visitors; whether the visitor is known to the students or not; whether the visitor is from inside or outside the institution; how the visitor is presented by the teacher. Most important, perhaps, is the role the observer takes in the session. Supervising tutors, for example, may insist on a non-participatory role to increase their objectivity, or a participatory one to diminish the effect of the scrutinizing assessor at the back of the classroom everyone is desperately trying to pretend doesn't exist! The important thing is for both the observer and observed teacher to be clear about their respective roles and the relationship between them. This will of course be, to some extent, predetermined. A line manager or a supervising tutor, however they may wish to play this down, have a supervisory, evaluative dimension to their role which a peer does not.

Figure 2.6 Three models of mentoring

The apprenticeship model	This notion is of a teacher working alongside an experienced professional, observing but also collaborating.
The competency model	Here, the mentor takes on the role of 'systematic trainer' or coach, with a predetermined list of competencies to tick off.
The reflective model	The mentor helps the teacher to develop a deeper understanding of student learning by joining them as co-enquirer.

Source: Maynard and Furlong 1993: 78–83.

The development of mentoring as a process in teacher education has grown largely as a result of the increase in school-based training in the last five or six years, as well as becoming widespread in industry and commerce. It is a practice which is now developing in PCE. Maynard and Furlong (1993) make a distinction between three models of mentoring which might usefully be applied to the relationship between observer and observed. The three models are shown in Figure 2.6.

Task 2.8

2.8(a) List those who have already and may in future be observing you teach: colleague, line manager, course tutor, mentor. Try to describe how you think they see their role as an observer.

2.8(b) If possible, present this view to them and ask them if this is, in fact, the way they do see their role. Were there discrepancies? If so, how do you account for these? How can they be minimized?

An effective relationship between observer and observed will involve an awareness of what the observer's focus will be, in the same way that you are aware of your own evaluation focus (see Task 2.4). Below are the aspects of communication skills and techniques the observer of the self-evaluation session in Section 2.3 chose to focus on:

• giving instructions, checking understanding;
• supporting pair work: keeping a balance between enabling and spoon-feeding;
• managing attending to individuals while monitoring the group;
• effective explanation of complex points;
• appropriate use of visual aids.

In considering observation, Wragg (1994) distinguishes between quantit-

Task 2.9

2.9(a) Describe to your partner a lesson you have recently given or soon will give, detailing both student and teacher activities.

2.9(b) Your partner should then select a focus for his or her observation of that lesson spelling out the features they intend to focus on. They should share these with you. How far did you or would you emphasize these features in your own self-evaluation?

ative and qualitative methods. The former represent an attempt to quantify aspects of lessons such as verbal interaction, the use of teaching aids and classroom management as a basis for evaluation. As Wragg points out, there are many ways in which such methods can be useful and he gives examples such as an observer wanting to know how many students get to use computer equipment or the length of answers students give to questions. But such systematic analysis, as we have seen, is more suited to a competency model of mentoring. And, although, as Wragg says, 'Quantitative and qualitative approaches need not be seen as polar opposites as they can often complement each other' (p. 10) it is likely that a qualitative approach with its focus on the nature of the learner's experience will be more helpful to a Certificate of Education student used to a more reflective model of evaluation.

We noted above that, although observation provided a more objective approach to evaluation than perhaps the teacher's own review, this is complicated by the observer's interpretation of events in the classroom, central to qualitative methods of observation. This interpretation will be influenced by a number of factors about the observers themselves:

- their background, experience and educational ideology;
- their awareness of and attitude to the lesson's subject/topic;
- their understanding of student responses, interactions and behaviour;
- their knowledge of and attitude to the teacher;
- their perception of their role and purpose as an observer;
- the way(s) in which they've recorded their observations.

Task 2.10

2.10(a) Table 2.1 shows a series of classroom events. On a scale of 1–5, where 5 means 'good practice' and 1 means 'bad practice', rate each event.

2.10(b) Would you give each the same rating if the subject of the session, where given, were different?

It is possible that there was disagreement over rating between members of the group. It is likely that you needed to know a great deal more about

Table 2.1 Evaluating classroom events

Classroom event	1	2	3	4	5
1 Students talk frequently in a session when they're working in small groups					
2 Students are free to move around the room					
3 The teacher gives a lecture lasting 40 minutes of the hour-long session, leaving 20 minutes for question and answer					
4 Most basic skills students' work is in small groups around tables					
5 The whiteboard is the main visual aid in a lecture					
6 All teaching is one-to-one or pair instruction in a sub-aqua class					
7 Students extensively assess one another's work in a business studies class					
8 The session is based exclusively on active learning – in this case games and role-play on a management course					
9 Students are involved mainly in recording information in a biology class					
10 The second year degree session is a seminar where one student reads a paper and the lecturer and students discuss it					

the context of the lesson before making a judgement. Even then, however, it is possible that group members actually sitting through the lesson itself might have reached different conclusions about what was happening and its value.

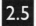 **2.5** *The context for your professional learning*

> KEY ISSUES
>
> The group is seen by many students to be their most important resource
>
> Experiencing a very different teaching context from your own can be as useful as experiencing a very similar one

You may be following a course of study either on your own or in small groups through distance learning. Many Certificate of Education groups, however, comprise a wide cross-section of practitioners and students and in their evaluations often cite the group they've been a part of as a (and often the) most important learning resource they've had access to. How can we make the best use of such a group for our professional development? The opportunity to carry out peer observations has already been considered in Section 2.4 and those of you who have completed a C&G 730 or similar course will be familiar with micro- or peer-group teaching and the opportunity it gives to practise skills in a secure and supportive environment. Below, however, are other ways in which Certificate of Education students have used group members and their professional contexts:

- developing and planning jointly-run courses;
- developing new resources, particularly course materials;
- conducting trials with one another's course materials;
- trying out teaching and learning strategies seen on peer observation sessions;
- team teaching with one another's groups.

Your response to these possibilities may be to throw up your hands in despair at the narrow specialism you teach. Clearly, there are important ways in which teachers sharing a subject area can collaborate. But it is surprising how much you can learn from areas which at first seemed so different from your own. Indeed, so isolated are many of us working in PCE that for those of you undertaking a course of professional training, such experience of diverse contexts is imperative.

Task 2.11: Working with others

2.11(a)   Each group member should give a brief account to the rest of the group of their professional context, as described earlier in Task 2.3.

2.11(b)   Now select three or four individual contexts you feel it might be useful to explore and, with each colleague, specify at least one way you might collaborate.

2.11(c)   Feed this back to the rest of the group
(2.11c often sparks even more ideas and possibilities).

2.6 *Assignment research and writing*

KEY ISSUES

Many students new to formal study find particular difficulty with essay/assignment writing

Practical advice includes:

- ensuring you answer the question asked
- engaging in systematic planning and research
- making at least one draft
- observing appropriate written conventions, including referencing and a bibliography

During your course you will be asked to present your work in a variety of oral and written forms: a jointly-authored piece of research or course design; a seminar presentation; a diary or reflective log; a workshop presentation. However, our own experience with students new to formal study, or returning to it after a considerable break, is that it is the written, discursive assignment or essay they find most difficulty with, and we shall therefore concentrate on this form of presentation here.

A common error made by students new to assignment writing is the tendency to include everything they know about a topic rather than answer the question they've been asked.

Task 2.12: Answering the question

2.12(a) Below is a series of assignment questions about the same assessment topic. Choose one of these titles and attempt, in one or two sentences, to outline what an appropriate answer might be.

2.12(b) Share your outlines with the group. Were there variations between answers?

1 Outline three assessment techniques you use and explain your reasons for using them.
2 Describe three assessment techniques you use and evaluate their effectiveness.
3 Compare and contrast three assessment techniques you use with respect to the kinds of student learning they measure.
4 Choose three assessment techniques you use and consider how positive student reaction is to them.
5 Analyse three assessment techniques you use and discuss the extent to which they measure what you say they do.

The key in Task 2.12 is to focus first on the verbs ('analyse', 'discuss', 'compare and contrast'), then on the nouns which form their objects. Question 1 asks for an outline of your strategies but then wants you to explain your reasons for using them. This part of the question invites quite a wide response: you may feel the strategies will measure the kind of learning you want; or that they're easy to use; or they may be pre-scribed by the syllabus. Question 2 is arguably more focused, requiring you to concentrate on the techniques' effectiveness, their validity, or the extent to which they measure what they say they do, as does Question 5, which also wants you to analyse the techniques rather than just describe them; that is, break them down into their component parts or elements. Question 3 wants you to concentrate on comparing and contrasting, in this case, different kinds of student learning, whereas Question 4 is more interested in student response or attitude.

Figure 2.7 Spider diagram in response to Question 2

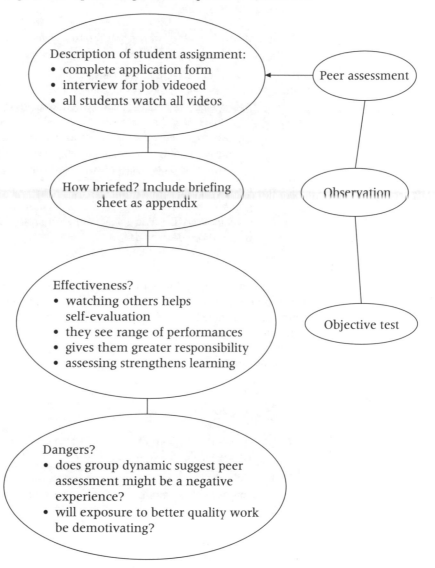

Once you feel clearer about what the assignment title is looking for, it is time to begin the planning and research process. A useful first stage is to pool your ideas (brainstorm) and record this on a spider diagram. Figure 2.7 shows a sample spider diagram for Question 2 with one strategy, Peer Assessment, broken down into sub-topics.

Organizing your ideas into a spider diagram helps you explore more than one way of structuring your assignment at the next stage, the assignment plan.

Task 2.13: Planning

2.13(a) Below is a series of approaches to answering Question 2. Which would be most effective?

1 In the first section, describe each assessment technique then, in the second, evaluate the effectiveness of each.
2 Describe the first technique, then evaluate it, the second, then evaluate it, and so on.
3 Take each element of effective assessment (e.g. objectivity/subjectivity, reinforcement of learning, ease of operation, validity, reliability) and consider particular techniques as they are relevant.

2.13(b) Compare your views with other members of the group. Would group members be more comfortable with one approach rather than another? Did you think of any other approaches in addition to the three described?

You are now ready for some targeted research. There may be something to be said for a wider, more scattergun approach to research at the brainstorming stage but you will soon see that the sheer volume of material available on most major post-compulsory issues makes this time consuming and of limited value. The chief resources for your targeted research are shown in Figure 2.8.

Task 2.14: Access to resources

2.14(a) As individuals, then as a group, which of the resources shown in Figure 2.8 do you have access to?

2.14(b) Consider how you may go about getting access to those resources not currently available to you as a group.

Depending on the number and extent of assignments, many tutors are happy to look at drafts. If not, you should certainly attempt at least one draft before submitting your final draft. Elements of the draft to consider are:

- Are you demonstrating an understanding of the issues you're dealing with? Have you dealt comprehensively with the subject and covered the breadth of topics required?
- Have you looked at topics in sufficient depth?
- Does your draft have balance: have you concentrated overmuch on one topic to the exclusion of others equally as important?
- Have you illustrated your points with examples? In making a case or developing an argument, it is not enough simply to *state* points – you

Figure 2.8 Resources for targeted research

Textbooks

Newspapers (particularly the *Times Educational Supplement*, the *Times Higher Educational Supplement* and other educational supplement and feature sections)

The internet (see specifically Section 5.6 on 'Newsgroups' in Chapter 5)

TV programmes

The experience of teaching colleagues

The experience of students

The experience of group members

Educational journals, particularly:

Adults Learning

Assessment in Education – principles, policy and practice

British Journal of Education and Work

Comparative Education

Curriculum Studies – a journal of education discussion and debate

Educa – the digest for vocational education and training

FE Now

General Education

Journal of Further and Higher Education

Studies in Higher Education

Teaching in Higher Education

should provide *support* for them. This could be done with evidence or arguments from the literature, the use of authorities or the experience of relevant parties.

- Have you used your reading appropriately? It is a mistake to quote chunks out of books and hope they'll speak for you. References should be relevant to what you want to say.
- Have you used written conventions appropriately? These may vary from course to course but tutors normally want to see assignments written in continuous prose. A common error is to write in note form or in some other abbreviated style using bullet points, letters or numerals. Sub-headings should only be used for longer pieces of work.

There are several systems of referencing but perhaps the most straightforward (and the one used in this book) is the Harvard system. This is based on author and date of publication. In the text, you should use the author's surname and the year of publication, e.g.:

. . . Bell (1987) argues that . . .

or:

'Finding information in the first place can be hard enough. Finding it again some time afterwards can be even harder unless your methods of recording and filing are thorough and systematic' (Bell 1987: 33).

In the bibliography, all books and articles consulted, read and referred to should be listed in alphabetical order, with author's name and initial followed by the date of publication, the title and finally the place of publication and the publisher. Thus, for this chapter, the bibliography would be set out as follows:

Bell, J. (1987) *Doing Your Research Project*. Milton Keynes: Open University Press.

Bloom, B.S. (1964) *Taxonomy of Educational Objectives: Handbook 1: Cognitive Domain*. London: Longman.

Gibbs, G., Habeshaw, S. and Habeshaw, T. (1988) *53 Interesting Ways to Appraise Your Teaching*. Bristol: Technical and Educational Services Ltd.

Maynard, T. and Furlong, J. (1993) Learning to teach and models of mentoring, in D. McIntyre, H. Hagger and M. Wilkin (eds) *Mentoring: Perspectives on School-based Teacher Education*. London: Kogan Page.

Wragg, E.C. (1994) *An Introduction to Classroom Observation*. London: Routledge.

Youngman, M.B. (1986) *Analysing Questionnaires*. Nottingham: University of Nottingham School of Education.

Judith Butcher's *Copy-Editing* (1992, 3rd edn, Cambridge University Press) gives a detailed guide to using the Harvard system.

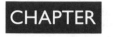

STUDENT LEARNING IN POST-COMPULSORY EDUCATION

What is Chapter 3 about?

'Learning' is the buzz-word that heralds the new millennium. We live in a 'learning society', where 'lifelong learning' has replaced a lifelong job; we work in 'learning organizations' and shop in the 'learning market' (DfEE 1995b), spending our individual learning accounts in order to fulfil our 'lifetime learning promise' (Barber 1996). The traditional distinction between education and training has been obscured by this new focus on learning. Does it mean that 'skills' and 'knowledge' are no longer viable concepts in a new era of 'learning'? Does 'learning' mean inclusiveness and a sweeping away of the old education/training divide? Indeed, the Department for Education and Employment (DfEE) consultative document, *Lifetime Learning* (1995b) suggests that in many cases the word 'training' has been replaced by 'learning' and that learning is for everyone. The report goes on to say that:

> Creating a culture of lifetime learning is crucial to sustaining and maintaining our international competitiveness. Technological change will dominate the working lifetimes of those now in work and we must be in a position to adapt. At the individual level, our personal competitiveness will have a major effect on our prosperity.
>
> (DfEE 1995b: 1.1)

So how does what appears to be an obsession with 'learning' relate to our students and what goes on in our classrooms? How does this changing understanding of what education, training, skills, knowledge and learning are, influence practice? Chapter 1 provided the context for understanding the changes in the post-compulsory sector and traced historical developments. This chapter seeks to develop your knowledge and understanding of selected theoretical perspectives in relation to current developments.

This chapter will explore key features of different learning theories in relation to classroom practice. Section 3.2 will examine the factors affecting students' ability to learn. What are the differences and similarities between a class of 17-year-old hairdressers, an adult education French class and a group of postgraduate student teachers? What affects a student's ability to learn? We will look critically at some of the factors that have particular contemporary significance. Section 3.3 will introduce some of the theories of learning as a background to our understanding of how our students learn. How have behaviourist, cognitive and humanist ideas about learning in particular affected approaches to teaching and learning? Section 3.4 will consider what constitutes effective learning and how barriers to learning can be overcome. Are we concerned with knowledge and understanding or with skills development? We will look at how we can ensure that our students learn effectively through an understanding of their learning styles and needs. How effective study skills and learner autonomy can be developed provides the focus for Section 3.5. What is the value and role of independent learning both within the classroom and as directed self-study? How is independent learning best managed and organized? These are the questions we will reflect upon and try to answer.

Factors affecting student learning

KEY ISSUES

What makes one group of learners distinct from another?

What individual differences can we identify in learners?

How can knowledge of factors which affect learning inform our approach to teaching?

Task 3.1

3.1(a) Choose one of your groups of learners and write a short profile of it giving details of what you know about individuals.

3.1(b) Look at what you have written and identify some general headings for the information you have included; for example ability, motivation, social background.

3.1(c) Now think about a contrasting group, preferably one that you teach, or alternatively one that you have been a student in recently – perhaps a tutor training group or adult education class. Write a similar profile using the headings you identified for your first group. What are the differences? What are the similarities? Note these down to return to later. You may like to discuss your observations with a colleague.

Strong claims are made for the distinctiveness of particular groups of learners. Indeed, a whole body of theory has been developed around the adult learner as distinct from younger learners. But what makes one group of learners distinct from another? Is it a question of age, motivation, ability, the chosen course of study? Every learning group is obviously different because it is made up of different individuals. Given the diverse nature of PCE you no doubt encounter a very wide variety of abilities, personalities, backgrounds and so on, among your students. These differences not only affect your approach to teaching, which will be considered in Chapter 4, but also have a marked effect on how students learn.

Task 3.2

3.2(a) Here is a list of factors which affect a student's ability to learn. It is not exhaustive and you may want to add others. In your experience, are any of these factors more important than others? Place them in order of importance.

- Ability
- Motivation
- Personality
- Attitude
- Age
- Learning style
- Home life
- Previous learning experience
- Life experience

3.2(b) Why do you consider some factors more important than others? Do some of them overlap?

3.2(c) Now look at each factor in turn and write down an example of how learning is enhanced and how it is inhibited in each case. For example, an older student may bring to a class a great deal of previous experience and knowledge on which they can build; on the other hand, they may be anxious about having had a long period away from education and because of their age have less confidence in their ability to learn.

The order of importance and examples that one chooses will depend to some extent on who the learners are and what they are learning, but there are commonalities as well as distinctive features. Continuity of educational experience is an important influence on the way people approach learning. The 16–19-year-old in FE and the traditional HE cohort has a continuous experience of education from at least the age of five. Schooling in one form or another has been a dominant feature of their lives. The routines and expectations of educational establishments are familiar to them. This is not generally the case for the adult learner who may not have been involved in a formal educational experience for some time and whose knowledge and expectations of education may only be based on their own school experience. Equally, the adult re-entering the education system at whatever level has many more outside responsibilities and pressures than the younger FE or HE student. That is not to play down the increased financial burdens that younger students now face in respect of tuition fees and the pressure to earn a living while studying, but these, and other pressures, are much more acute for the adult 'returner'. We shall consider these issues in more detail in Section 3.4 in the context of barriers to learning.

Social and political contexts are important influences on the way teaching and learning are approached and the relative importance given to one theoretical perspective over another. For example, the issues of ability, motivation and ageing might be considered to have particular significance at the present time given the nature of the current preoccupation with education and the new political emphasis on lifetime learning. Let us look at these three factors in more detail with a contemporary focus.

Ability

Ability, and more specifically, intelligence, is perhaps the most contentious and politicized aspect of learning. Even a commonly accepted definition has been elusive. Nor have approaches to measuring intelligence and establishing the intelligence quotient (IQ) of individuals been consensual. Is intelligence fixed? What are the relative influences of heredity and social circumstances on an individual's intelligence? Does IQ exist at all? Can intelligence be measured? These questions remain unresolved.

Attempts at the description and definition of intelligence have often focused on the differences between individuals. Those perceived differences have then often been used for political ends. Take for example the eugenics movement in the early part of the twentieth century whose aim it was to 'improve' the human race. Drawing on Darwin's theories of evolution as they could be applied to society (social Darwinism) and theories of heredity and genetic influences current at that time, eugenicists essentially claimed a scientific basis for white Anglo-Saxon superiority. These theories gave a justification not just to the sort of 'master race' ideas of Nazi Germany, but had already led to numerous pieces of legislation in the United States between 1911 and 1930. Laws were passed in some states allowing for the sterilization of 'misfits', the 'mentally retarded' and the 'insane' and to restrict marriages between certain racial groups.

Eugenics has since been discredited. And yet its spectre seems to stalk present research into genetics and IQ. Nowadays, there is general unease about aspects of genetic research from an ethical point of view. For example, the search for genes which might influence variations in intelligence is viewed with scepticism not for the scientific data researchers present, but for the implications of their findings and the uses they might be put to. What if it were true, as some scientists claim, that genetic factors account for 50 per cent of IQ variations across the population? What might be the effect of such a claim on the way teachers view their students?

Other recent research claims that genetic make-up as much as the socialization process dictates differences between boys and girls in terms of how they acquire social skills, suggesting that gender differences are largely genetically rather than culturally determined (Skuse 1997). What are the implications of such claims? At the present time, there seems to be a certain coyness about research into genes and IQ perhaps due to the fear of a backlash. In a more confident age this was not the case.

> **Task 3.3**
>
> What examples can you draw on (either from observation of students, your own children or others around you) that appear to be inherited traits? Can you identify any social influence – that is, aspects of upbringing, peer influences or the wider influences in society – that might give an alternative explanation for any of these traits?

The 'nature-nurture' discussion has been a subject of research and debate among scientists and educationalists throughout the twentieth century. Intelligence testing is an attempt to identify the innate ability of the individual. Intelligence tests were first developed at the turn of the century in France by Binet and Simon. Under contract to the French government, their task was to devise a test to identify children who should benefit from special schooling. This test was adapted in the United States and in 1916 became widely known as the Stanford-Binet test (see Child 1993: 210–12). It has been used widely, in modified forms, to measure normal, subnormal and superior intelligence throughout the century. In Britain, the work of Cyril Burt is perhaps the best-known in the field. Burt's theories formed the whole basis of accepted wisdom on the nature of intelligence for generations of schoolchildren from the 1950s onward. He established that intelligence was partly innate and partly developed as a result of the social environment. His theories were adopted and resulted in the 11+ examination and IQ testing in schools. In later years Burt was criticized for his deterministic approach, and more recently it has been suggested that he falsified some of his data (Hearnshaw 1979).

Since the 1960s, social and cultural factors have been considered more important determinants of intelligence than heredity. While individual differences in ability are acknowledged, educators have regarded social inequalities as influencing more profoundly an individual's capacity for learning. The abandonment (in most parts of the country) of the 11+ examination in the early 1970s was the ideological expression of an attempt at engineering a more egalitarian society through the education system. The value of IQ tests as they were conceived of in the 1950s and 1960s was called into question on the basis that they were gender and culturally biased, aimed at middle-class children who generally performed better and were not an accurate measure of ability for most people.

The 'nature-nurture' debate usually centres on the relative importance of heredity over social factors, but it is also worth taking a step back and asking the question: does IQ actually exist? From as long ago as the beginning of the nineteenth century it has been argued in some quarters that the nature of intelligence cannot be coded, certainly not genetically coded, and that intelligence by its nature has no limitations and is not parcelled-out in specific amounts. Nor is it a merely abstract potential; rather, it has a real and determinant content. It is well known that concentrated teaching can improve IQ scores and that generation by generation IQ scores are improving. What does this tell us? It might also be argued that IQ has served the role of justifying social inequalities in that we live in a meritocracy where income is distributed according to merit and merit is defined as intelligence plus effort. Could it be that the elevation of intelligence as a defining factor of success or failure in society is a way of endorsing social divisions?

Task 3.4

3.4(a) Individual differences in ability clearly have an impact on our approach to teaching. In what ways do you take the differing abilities of your learners into account in order to ensure that each individual achieves their potential?

3.4(b) If possible, compare your ideas with a partner and draw up a list together of how you *differentiate* your approach to teaching according to students' varying abilities.

Motivation

Motivation is a key factor in learning and is linked very closely to attitude. Motivation has been described as 'a person's aroused desire for participation in a learning process' (Curzon 1990: 195). How to arouse and maintain that desire is of concern both to the student and the tutor. Our students arrive in our classes with all sorts of motives for attending. Those motives may be positive and lead a student to be well motivated towards learning, or they may be somewhat negative leading a student to be poorly motivated towards learning.

At the present time the majority of young people continue their education beyond the age of 16. HE has expanded to accommodate a much more diverse student population including a larger proportion of mature students. Unemployed people of all ages are required to attend education and training courses. An increasing number of adults attend Adult Education Centres for more functional reasons than for the pleasure of learning for its own sake. These changes in our student population bring with them changes in student motives and motivation.

Task 3.5

3.5(a) Choose one of your teaching groups and find out (if you don't already know) what were their individual motives for attending your course.

3.5(b) Now consider how their initial motives for joining the course relate to their *attitudes to learning* during the course.

3.5(c) Can you identify any changes in attitudes as the course has progressed? How do you account for these changes?

Motivation is often seen as needs-related. Perhaps the most well-known theory of motivation is Maslow's hierarchy of needs (Maslow 1970: 56–61). Maslow, whose work is closely related to humanistic psychology saw 'self-actualization' as what drives people to learn; that is, the need to make full use of one's talents, become creative and achieve one's potential is what motivates us. Self-actualization is an ultimate human goal and need, but before that need can be fulfilled a set of other needs must be met. These needs are generally presented as a pyramid, shown in Figure 3.1. At the bottom level are physiological needs such as hunger and thirst. Once these are satisfied the next level is the need for physical and psychological well-being which if met leads on to the need for love and a sense of belonging which involves having warm, friendly relationships. Next come self-esteem needs: to achieve, be successful, have the respect of others. Finally, at the top of the hierarchy is self-actualization, the desire to fulfil one's potential. This, according to Maslow may only be achieved by some people fleetingly throughout their lives, but the top of the pyramid is left open because human potential is not finite. The important thing to recognize about Maslow's hierarchy is that moving to a higher level is dependent on the level below. It follows therefore that a self-actualized person can only become so if all the other needs are met. Can you identify these characteristics among the students you teach? Is it true, as Maslow seems to imply, that only well-off people in caring relationships and successful in their lives can achieve their full creative potential and self-fulfilment? And if so, what are the implications of this theory in relation to your students?

Maslow has been criticized for basing his theories on middle-class

Figure 3.1 Maslow's hierarchy of needs

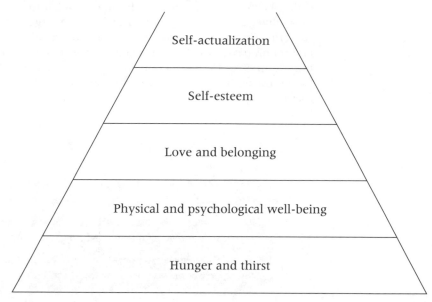

Self-actualization

Self-esteem

Love and belonging

Physical and psychological well-being

Hunger and thirst

Source: Maslow 1970.

America in the 1960s. Lessons from history as well as our own experience as teachers and learners tell us that it is not necessarily the case that motivation to learn is dependent on the fulfilment of interrelated needs in the hierarchical way that Maslow describes. Equally, the extent to which the tutor can meet certain of those needs may be limited. But what aspects of Maslow's theory are relevant to learners in PCE?

Task 3.6

3.6(a) Take each stage of Maslow's hierarchy of needs and consider what the practical implications are for your teaching. For example, *love and belonging* might be interpreted in the classroom as creating a positive, supportive atmosphere.

3.6(b) How will each of these practical considerations enhance student motivation?

Other theorists such as Robert Gagné have identified motivation as the first phase of the learning process. The role of the teacher, according to Gagné, is 'to identify the motives of students and channel them into activities that accomplish educational goals' (1977: 206). It is essential to student motivation that the teacher identifies and communicates goals and objectives to students and generates expectations in them. What effect do low expectations on the part of the tutor and the student have on student motivation? Is it more a problem today when students may have limited career prospects and may have chosen to continue in education and training because there was no alternative in a dwindling labour market?

Task 3.7

3.7(a) Note down what strategies you use to promote and maintain the motivation of your students.

3.7(b) Compare your strategies with a partner's. What are the similarities and differences? How do you account for these?

Intrinsic and *extrinsic* are other descriptions that have been applied to motivation. Intrinsic motivation is said to come from an inner drive and this is related to the human need for self-esteem and self-confidence and a desire to satisfy curiosity. Some activities are a reward in themselves and undertaken purely for the pleasure they give. Extrinsic motivation on the other hand is externally produced. Some external incentive with some sort of promise of reward, threat of punishment or need for competition or cooperation with others characterizes this type of motivation. For extrinsic motivation to be sustained, students must have attainable goals to work towards, be given immediate feedback on their performance and be rewarded for success. It is fashionable nowadays to focus more on developing an atmosphere of cooperation among students and eliminating any sort of competitive spirit in the classroom as this is seen as being harmful to students, particularly the low achievers. However, competitiveness is linked with achievement and doing one's best. Is it possible that the effect of discouraging competition is to damage motivation and ultimately the fulfilment of individual aspiration and potential?

Cyril Houle (1961) provides a similar description of motivation in what he calls the 'orientation of learning' of students, and identifies three types of learner. First, the *goal-orientated* learner who engages in a course for specific reasons with clear objectives such as obtaining a qualification, completing a task or project or solving an immediate problem. Once the objective has been achieved this type of learner generally ceases to attend her or his course of study. Second, the *activity-orientated* learner who joins a class because they enjoy the social engagement that learning offers as well as the course content. This type of learner feels as much benefit from being a part of a group as acquiring new skills or knowledge and returns year after year moving from one course to another. If you work in an AE setting, this type of learner may be familiar to you. The third type of orientation Houle calls *learning-orientated*. This type of learner enjoys learning for its own sake and attends a course purely out of interest in the subject. Such a learner may continue to study alone long after the course has finished to extend their knowledge further.

Task 3.8

3.8(a) Can you think of examples of how your learners are motivated intrinsically and extrinsically? How do these examples relate to Houle's 'orientations of learning'?

3.8(b) Discuss in a small group the relative merits of cooperation and competition in enhancing motivation. Are they mutually exclusive? What might be the effects on learning of entirely eradicating the one or the other in the classroom?

Ageing

The achievement of individual potential as a lifelong goal seems a laudable aspiration. No longer is it the case that age, in theory at any rate, is seen as a barrier to access to education. We have national training targets which aim to train 60 per cent of the adult workforce up to NVQ Level 3 or equivalent by the year 2000 (HMSO 1995). It is now clearly understood that the opportunity to continue learning throughout life is part of what it means to be a mature, healthy adult.

The present-day understanding of adult learning is partly based on psychological lifespan development theories which date from the late 1960s. Up to that time it was assumed that once people had achieved biological maturity their ability to learn became 'stable' – that is, reached a plateau – and then began to deteriorate. This is called the *decrement model* of adult development. Research undertaken subsequently by a number of academics have concluded that this is not the case. The *personal growth model* which now has general currency presents ageing in a less negative light, stressing positive aspects of human development. Several similar descriptive inventories of 'phases' or 'stages' of the human life cycle are available (Tennant 1988). For example Chickering and Havighurst (1981) in the United States drew on the empirical work of others (and earlier work by Havighurst) to construct an 'inventory of life': Developmental Tasks of the Adult Years. They identified six phases in the adult life cycle related to chronological ages, as follows. Late adolescence and youth (16–23) is characterized by an emphasis on achieving emotional independence, choosing and preparing for a career, preparing for marriage and family life and developing an ethical system. Early adulthood (23–35) focuses on deciding on a partner, starting a family, managing a home, starting in an occupation and assuming a civic occupation. Mid-life transition (35–45) is a period of adapting to a changing time perspective, revising career plans and redefining family relationships. Middle adulthood (45–57) is concerned with maintaining a career or developing a new one, restabilizing family relationships, making mature civic contributions and adjusting to biological change. Late adult transition (57–65) is a period of preparation for retirement and in late adulthood (65+) the individual is adjusting to retirement, adjusting to declining health and strength, becoming affiliated with late-adult age groups, establishing satisfactory living arrangements, adjusting to the death of a spouse and maintaining integrity.

You may consider that Chickering and Havighurst's model is somewhat prescriptive and bears little resemblance to the lives of many people in present-day society. Indeed, one of the criticisms of their work and that of others in a similar vein is that their descriptions tended to be based on middle-class white American males at a particular time in history.

Task 3.9

3.9(a) Discuss in a small group what would be the objections to the above description of adult development. How might such a model be useful to you?

3.9(b) What sort of 'inventory of life' might apply to your students?

However, while criticisms are levelled at aspects of lifespan development theories, there is nevertheless a general professional acceptance that adulthood is a period of change and development and that in principle, an adult's capacity to learn throughout life is not significantly diminished. However, it may not be generally acknowledged amongst the general public that this is the case. How often do our adult students use their age as an excuse for some difficulty they have with their learning?

Task 3.10

3.10(a) List all the difficulties with learning something that your students (or you!) have attributed to their age.

3.10(b) Which ones have a physical cause and which ones might be caused by other factors (e.g. social)?

3.10(c) Discuss in a group ways of helping your students overcome these difficulties.

The demographic reality of an ageing population has contributed to some extent to changes in attitudes to age and ageing. After all, by the year 2001 16 per cent of the population in Britain will be over the age of 64 and by 2041 this figure will reach 25 per cent. In a general sense the old cliché 'You can't teach an old dog new tricks' is no longer credible, although at an individual level, as we have seen, many people lack confidence in their ability to learn as they get older.

It is not surprising that ageing is a preoccupation of the 1990s since an increasingly ageing population is assumed to be a burden on society. Whether or not this is the case is disputed since there is little evidence to support the assertion. However, it is clearly in the interests of society to keep as much of the population as possible active and healthy for as long as possible in order to reduce the effects of that perceived burden.

An alternative to the lifespan development theories is to see adult development as a dialectical process; that is, the change and development of the individual is both a product of the change and development of society and the agent of change and development in that society. This approach to understanding adulthood rejects psychological explanations of adult development. Rather, it is argued, the development of the individual is governed by the objective circumstances of their lives. If opportunities to learn, achieve and develop potential are restricted then the potential to learn will eventually become restricted. 'Use it or lose it' is the old adage. The extent to which society can enable everyone to achieve their potential is a perennial discussion and raises the issue of whether education should be for the benefit of the individual or the greater benefit of society. In the context of our discussion of ageing and learning, it is clear that the extent to which people have the opportunity to be physically and mentally active and to fulfil individual potential is important at all ages and is no less of a priority for the elderly.

In practical terms, however, we know that some older learners do experience certain physical difficulties such as hearing, sight and mobility. The important thing to remember is that these difficulties do not necessarily signal an impaired ability to learn. As you identified in Task 3.10, they merely require fairly straightforward changes of approach to learning both on the part of the tutor and the learner.

Task 3.11

Discuss with a partner some of the difficulties you have come across with older students. What strategies have you used or could you use to overcome them?

3.3   *Learning theories*

KEY ISSUES

What are the main theoretical perspectives that inform our approach to learning?

How does an understanding of theories of learning affect our approach to classroom practice?

It is not the intention here to provide an in-depth study of learning theories, but to present an overview of the main theoretical perspectives and to raise some critical issues related to them. Since the whole chapter is devoted to learning, aspects of theory are presented throughout and relate to the schools of thought discussed in this section. Theories of learning are based on psychological understanding and seek to describe what happens when learning takes place. Learning theory in essence is not about the conditions required for effective learning: it is for the practitioner to extract and interpret elements from theories and apply what is perceived as relevant to his or her own teaching. No one theory can supply a blueprint for how we learn, but each offers insights which are essential to us as teachers if we are to ensure that our students learn effectively.

All too often textbooks on educational psychology and learning theory, while explaining clearly the principles of learning, are less effective in the practical advice they give. As Tight (1996: 24) suggests, they offer a '"cook book" approach to practical advice'. This is because they do not relate to the content of the learning that is to be undertaken, but to the process of learning. The application of learning theory should therefore proceed on this basis; some insights into how people learn seem more appropriately applied to certain areas of subject matter than others, as we shall examine.

The broad strands of learning theory are: Behavourism, Gestalt theories, Cognitive Theories and Andragogy. Behaviourist, Gestalt and Cognitive Theories of learning have tended to centre round how learning occurs in children and date from the latter part of the nineteenth century. Andragogy and related theories, concerned with how adults learn as distinct from young people, are more recent and derive from the Humanist school of psychology.

According to Behaviourist theories, which formed the basis for all learning theories, all behaviour is learned, thus eliminating any biological influences. Put crudely, behaviourists contended that all learning involves 'an observable change in behaviour' and only what can be measured can be regarded as learning. Behaviourist psychologists did not seek to discover anything about thought processes, but about how learning occurred. Experiments involving salivating dogs (Classical Conditioning, after Pavlov), cats and monkeys (the Law of Effect, after Thorndike), rats and pigeons (Operant Conditioning, after Skinner) are well known and are the basis of S-R (Stimulus-Response) theory. The earliest behaviourist was Watson who established the principle of Trial and Error learning which other behaviourists developed. For a full account of individuals' work in this field see Child (1993: 92–9). The American psychologist B.F. Skinner has been perhaps the most influential figure in the field. Skinner developed some of the main principles by which behaviourist theory is known (1938). His 'Skinner box' involved putting hungry rats into a box and 'training' them to pull a series of levers to release food pellets. At first, pulling the lever was accidental, but after it happened several times, the rat began to associate pulling the lever with food and then did so intentionally, thus displaying learned behaviour. Such behaviour he called operant conditioning and what differentiates it from classical conditioning is that the individual is required to act on the environment (the rat operated the lever to obtain the food). The need for reinforcement, rewards and punishment and feedback are all attributable to Skinner's work. Skinner's experiments with teaching pigeons to walk in a figure of eight led to his identifying these elements as key features of learning: correct responses are reinforced by rewards, incorrect responses are ignored (or possibly punished, a negative reinforcement). Skinner subsequently made a major contribution to the development of programmed learning, the early fore-runner of computer-assisted learning and mastery learning. Skinner's Operant Conditioning also forms the basis of behaviour modification, the technique used to bring about a change in behaviour, often used in special needs education.

In a Behaviourist approach, learning should progress step-by-step and build on previously learned material. In the early stages the learner should be regularly rewarded when correct responses are given. This feedback stimulates motivation to continue. Learning is reinforced by rewards and knowledge of success. Skinner's work and the behaviourist method in general is appealing in that they identify components of learning which we can readily understand. Anyone who has trained a dog to sit on command or potty-trained a small child will recognize the features of the behaviourist method. But does *all* learning occur in this way? Essential to a behavioural view of learning is that any learning can be measured. Can all learning be observed? What about more abstract knowledge such as understanding Plato or appreciating classical music? Is there is a danger, therefore that anything that cannot be measured in behavioural terms gets ignored?

Task 3.12

3.12(a) Think of two examples from your own teaching where you could or do use a behaviourist approach. Describe how the learning takes place step-by-step.

3.12(b) Discuss your examples with a partner and try to apply the Behaviourist terminology to stages in the learning.

3.12(c) Draw up a list with your partner of the *types* of learning activity that might best be approached through behaviourist methods.

The examples you chose in Task 3.12 may well have been drawn from a vocational or competence-based course. For example, NVQs, which are discussed in various contexts elsewhere in this book offer the current exemplar of behaviourist theories of learning. Indeed, many professional qualifications, including the PGCE and the Certificate of Education are competence-based courses. If you write a lesson plan or course pro-gramme with objectives which state precisely what students will be able to do (for example, 'name the parts of the internal combustion engine'), you are writing behavioural objectives intending to measure a learning outcome. The competence movement has become perhaps the most important influence in the post-compulsory curriculum today.

The contribution of Gestalt psychology to learning is particularly important with regard to perception and the role it plays in learning. Wertheimer, Kohler and Koffler founded the Gestalt school of psychology in the 1920s. Unlike behaviourists who attempted to analyse behaviour, however complex, into stimulus-response units, Gestalt theory looks at how we see patterns as a whole. In fact, *Gestalt* means 'pattern' or 'form' in German. The visual 'trick' silhouette pictures which have two interpretations are well-known examples used to illustrate visual perception. The Gestaltists concluded from experiments such as these that the way we look at things and the ways in which we perceive things depends on our prior experience. They emphasized *closure*, which is our ability to process component parts of information and create a whole, and described this as *insight*. Insight learning applies the laws of perception to learning. It refers to that sudden flash of inspiration that we have when we suddenly see the solution to a problem. To experience what is meant by insight learning, try doing a jigsaw puzzle without the picture to guide you. You will proceed by trial and error, but at some stage, hopefully, you will have that sudden insight as to where to place a crucial piece as you realize what the picture is supposed to be. Insight, according to Gestaltists, is a response to a whole situation, not separate responses to a series of stimuli, as behaviourists would suggest. 'The whole is greater than the sum of its parts' is a description often applied to Gestalt theory, suggesting that something is missing in the Behaviourist approach. From a Gestalt perspective, learning is a complex process of interrelationships which occur as a result of engaging with a new problem in the light of previous experiences.

Task 3.13

3.13(a) What other examples of insight learning can you think of?

3.13(b) How does insight learning feature in *your* students' learning? Think of some examples.

Gestalt theories add another dimension to Behaviourism in terms of an understanding of learning processes. Insight learning and theories of perception are often described within the cognitive theoretical framework in study texts because they have in common an emphasis on more abstract psychological concepts such as 'understanding', 'reasoning', 'thinking' and 'human consciousness' as opposed to a simplistic attempt to reduce the rich variety of human learning to 'observable behaviour'. Piaget is the most well-known of the cognitive theorists writing and researching over a period of some forty years from the late 1920s to the early 1940s (see

Child 1993: 157–70). Although his work was focused on the development of children, he established nevertheless that learning is developmental. This has important implications for adult learning since it suggests that adulthood is a stable period in terms of intellectual development. Through experimentation, observation and research Piaget identified stages of intellectual development in children which are sequential and established that the changing nature of learning and the capacity to think throughout childhood is qualitative rather than quantitative. These developmental stages are known as: sensory motor (0–2 years); pre-operational (2–6 years); concrete operational (7–11 years); and formal operational (12 years +) (see Tennant 1988: 66–81 for a full account and critique in relation to adult learning). In short, each stage marks the development from practical thought to the abstract thought equated with mature adulthood. Is this an end point? Some theorists argue that it is not. Is the process necessarily age-related or more to do with the range and depth of learning experiences that we undergo at any age? Piaget has been criticized both for a lack of rigour in his methodology and for over-interpretation of his data. Nevertheless his analysis has been the bedrock of learning theory for a vast number of schoolteachers for the last 40 years or more (see Boden 1994).

A key feature of cognitive theory is that knowledge is constructed through interaction with the environment. It is a cognitive process which involves acquiring new information which enables the learner to evolve and transform their existing knowledge and then check out and apply the new state of knowledge to new situations; and so the process goes on. New patterns of meaning and understanding are formed to enable further learning to take place. The process is dynamic. The work of Jerome S. Bruner in the 1960s to 1980s, following on from and influenced by Piaget, has made a significant contribution to Cognitive Theory. For Bruner, it is essential that the learner has a fundamental understanding of the underlying principles of a subject. Discovery learning, according to Bruner, is the most effective and authentic method of achieving a real understanding of the principles of a subject and then applying those principles. Discovery learning involves confronting the learner with a problem and allowing them to explore the problem and try out solutions on the basis of inquiry and previous learning under the guidance of a teacher. The newly-acquired knowledge is then used to formulate a general principle which can then be applied to other situations. For example, when learning the concept of 'conservation' a young child might be given variously-shaped containers, a measuring jug and a bowl of water with which to 'play'. The child is encouraged by the teacher to try pouring water from one container to another. Some of the containers, although differently shaped, contain the same amount. Gradually through experimentation, and prompting and questioning by the teacher, the child arrives at an understanding that the quantity of water remains constant and is able to articulate her or his understanding. Over a period of time, he or she would be given further opportunities to demonstrate her or his knowledge and apply the principle in other situations.

Task 3.14

3.14(a) Discovery learning has been a popular approach with very young learners for the past 30 years or more. Discuss in a small group examples of how it might be an appropriate approach with learners in PCE.

3.14(b) Think of some examples from your own experience where you have encouraged discovery learning. Compare these examples with those from Task 3.15 below.

3.14(c) What would be the role of the teacher in a discovery learning situation?

David Ausubel, another cognitivist theorist, is critical of discovery learning. His work focused on what he called reception learning; that is, instruction. He emphasized the need for learning to be meaningful in that it should relate to the learner's existing knowledge. He advocated the straightforward exposition of a topic by the teacher as being more effective and less time-consuming than discovery learning.

Task 3.15

3.15(a) Think of examples from your own experience where reception learning is most appropriate. Compare these examples with those you identified for discovery learning.

3.15(b) What would be the role of the teacher in reception learning?

3.15(c) What do you think are the relative merits of reception learning over discovery learning?

Cognitive theorists relate their theories to subject content, as do behaviourists. The approach of humanist psychologists is more concerned with the process of learning and therefore contrasts sharply with behaviourism and cognitivism. Theories of learning related to humanistic psychology were arrived at as a reaction against Behaviourism and provide the intellectual basis for much adult learning theory. According to humanist insights, learning is a total personality process; life is a learning experience; true education is individual and about personal growth. Malcolm Knowles presents Andragogy, 'the science and art of helping adults to learn' (Knowles 1984: 52) as a theory of adult learning. It was Knowles who developed and popularized the andragogical model, the notions of the adult as a self-directed learner, and the 'learning contract'. Knowles based his model on his experiences in teaching in American universities which has been pointed to as an essential weakness of his theories. While

Table 3.1 The Assumptions of Andragogy

	Pedagogical	*Andragogical*
Concept of the learner	Dependent personality	Increasingly self-directed
Role of learner's experience	To be built on, more than used as a resource	A rich resource for learning by self and other
Reading to learn	Uniform by age, level and curriculum	Develops from life tasks and problems
Orientation to learning	Subject-centred	Task or problem-centred
Motivation	By external rewards and punishment	By internal incentives and curiosity

Source: Knowles 1984: 116.

the 'Assumptions of Andragogy' have been challenged and much criticized, nevertheless the notion of the self-directed learner underpins much of adult education practice and remains the keystone of adult learning theory. Many tutors working in FE colleges in particular are familiar with learning contracts which have been introduced in recent years. Knowles identified five elements of the learning process: the concept of the learner; the role of the learner's experience; readiness to learn; orientation to learning; and motivation. He contrasted a characterization of pedagogical assumptions with what he identified as andragogical. Table 3.1 sets out Knowles' 'assumptions'.

Task 3.16

Discuss in a group of four or five the extent to which you would support or reject the assumptions in Table 3.1. Use examples from your own experience of children and adults learning to inform your discussion.

Humanist psychologists, in particular Carl Rogers, provided a framework of understanding upon which Knowles built, rejecting previous theories of learning as being only appropriate to children. Rogers, a therapist, applied his observations of adults in therapy to learning and conceptualized student-centred learning as a parallel to his client-centred therapy. 'Teaching, in my estimation, is a vastly over-rated function' (Rogers 1983: 119). Rogers considered that the 'facilitation of learning' with a focus on the interpersonal relationship between the learner and the facilitator based on trust, 'empathic understanding' and genuineness on the part of the facilitator is the key to effective learning. 'Changingness, a reliance on *process* rather than upon static knowledge, is the only thing that makes any sense as a goal for education in the modern world' (1983: 120, original emphasis). According to Rogers, much significant learning is acquired by doing, and therefore experiential learning is the only true learning, and the antipathy of any sort of memory learning. Like Knowles, Rogers emphasizes the 'self', self-development and self-direction. Unlike Knowles, for whom 'self-direction' involves the learner controlling the *content* of a course according to their needs while the tutor controls the *processes*, Rogers leaves the process in the hands of the learner and content appears to have little importance. Rogers in common with Knowles, has been criticized for offering a partial theory, but both have nevertheless been very influential in the development of contemporary thinking on adult education.

Indeed, many of the ideas relating to andragogy and humanistic psychology have passed into a common-sense understanding of how learning is best 'facilitated' with learners in all sectors of PCE and are actively promoted by many mainstream educationalists. However, certain problems arise from the wholesale adoption of such an approach to teaching and learning. Tennant (1988: 23) provides a useful, if partial in itself, summary of his reservations concerning andragogy:

> ... I have argued that the rationale and empirical support for the humanistic concepts of self-development and self-direction has gaps and weaknesses which need to be acknowledged. There is a need to distinguish the rhetoric of adult education from its rationale and empirical base. The prevailing rhetoric asserts that in everyday life adults are basically self-directed and that this self-direction is rooted in our constitutional make-up, it also asserts that self-development is an inexorable process towards higher levels of existence, and finally it asserts that adult learning is fundamentally (and necessarily) different from child learning. These assertions should not be accepted as articles of faith.

Task 3.17

3.17(a) Reflect on your classroom practice and consider the ways in which theories of learning based on humanistic psychology have influenced your teaching.

3.17(b) Consider the issues raised in the paragraph above and discuss with a partner your ideas for dealing with them.

It is also useful to think about the consequences of elevating process over content, by replacing the *what* with the *how* in teaching and learning. Is self-direction the starting point or the goal of education? Does the practice of experiential learning reduce all learning to the functional? Is the transmission of knowledge and the pursuit of excellence redundant? What does it mean to be a 'facilitator of learning'?

3.4 *Effective learning*

KEY ISSUES

How do we identify learning needs and learning styles?

What are barriers to learning and how can they be overcome?

How do we help students to learn effectively?

Each group of learners is different from the next; each student is an individual with his or her own goals and expectations. These may or may not coincide with those of the tutor or the externally prescribed goals of a syllabus. A sound starting point for any course is to share those goals and where possible negotiate a consensus on what can be achieved by the group and by individuals in that group. It is often the case that some goals are predetermined by the nature of the course; preparation for achieving a qualification, for example. From the tutor's perspective, it is very useful to know what your students learning needs are, their motives for joining the course and so on in order to support their learning more effectively. What do students need to know about you and what you are going to teach them?

Task 3.18

3.18(a) List the information you need to know about your students and their learning needs, aspirations and expectations at the beginning of your course. Discuss your list with a partner and draw up a short questionnaire that you could use with your students.

3.18(b) Now think about the start of your course from a student's perspective. What information could you provide them with?

3.18(c) Why is this information exchange important? How can you use the information you obtain?

Of course not all students have a clear idea what their goals, expectations or aspirations are. Is it always possible or even legitimate within the confines of a prescribed programme of study in a group situation to expect to have all of one's individual, sometimes idiosyncratic needs met? However, by discussing these issues early on, it is possible to set a mutually supportive, cooperative tone to the course conducive to effective learning.

Do all learners approach their learning in the same way? Do individuals have a 'preferred style' of learning? Within the framework of experiential learning, several theorists have evolved models of learning styles. Perhaps the most well-known of these and the most frequently used with students is Kolb's (1984) 'learning style inventory'. Based on his model of experiential learning, David Kolb identified four categories of learning which occur in a cycle of concrete experience (CE), followed by observation and reflection on that experience (RO), then by the formulation of some sort of theory or hypothesis which involves abstract conceptualization (AC), and then, finally, by the testing-out of the hypothesis or theory in active experimentation (AE). According to Kolb the truly effective learner has abilities in all these four areas but most people have varying abilities in one area or another. The purpose of the inventory is to measure the relative strengths individuals have in each area by completing a questionnaire and then plotting the results on a quadrant. This enables the learner to identify her or his orientation to learning and discover how, given his or her natural inclinations, learning can best be approached. How useful is the method in identifying areas of 'weakness' and how might the information be used? There is an example recently of an individual who displayed the 'wrong' orientation to learning according to Kolb's inventory, and was refused entry onto a professional training course as a result.

Task 3.19

3.19(a) Consider what practical strategies might be employed to enhance student learning as a result of using Kolb's learning style inventory.

3.19(b) To what extent could or should such an exercise be used to assess learning needs? What other factors might be taken into account?

It is undoubtedly the case that people learn in different ways partly because they are different individuals and partly as a result of the subject matter on hand. It is important that the tutor has a clear understanding of what is to be learned in order to teach it effectively. If we are all individuals, all with our own learning styles, does that mean that we all need an individual learning programme? If that is the case, then what is the value of learning as a social activity? Would people gain more from learning alone in their own way?

Clearly, teaching methodology and course content need to be considered in relation to the learning styles of students. Discussion of appropriate methodology and classroom management issues can be found in Chapter 4. The task here has been to consider the role that learning styles have in relation to effective learning. If students are aware of their strengths and weaknesses in their approach to learning and are given consistent guidance by the tutor as to how they can build on their strengths and improve on their weaknesses, then they are more likely to have been successful in their studies. Robin Barrow (1984: 107) suggests that 'People come to learning in different ways, partly as a result of content, partly as a result of being different people preferring to or finding it easier to acquire understanding in different ways' and points to the importance of the relationship between how people learn and a clear understanding by the teacher of what is to be learned. Let us now turn to how effective learning can best be promoted.

We have already looked at various theoretical perspectives on learning, and the point has been made that learning is related to content. Any number of claims can be made about how learning is best achieved, but what is learned is the test of how effective the learning has been.

Let us consider a typical classroom scenario on a Certificate of Education course. The topic for the session is 'equal opportunities in PCE'. The sequence of the lesson is as follows:

1 Tutor 'brainstorms' ideas with students about what equal opportunities issues they have come across, either from their own experience or the experience of others.
2 Tutor gives a short talk about legislation and its impact/success/failure and invites the questions/comments/views of students.
3 In groups of four, students discuss various short case studies of practical equal opportunities issues and are asked to offer possible solutions to the problems.
4 Small groups feed back their ideas to the whole group.
5 Tutor leads group in a discussion of the underlying causes of inequality and draws together key points from the session.

Task 3.20

3.20(a) What are the strengths and weaknesses of the lesson? Look at each stage, preferably with a partner, and discuss how you would ensure that students learned effectively.

3.20(b) What is missing? For example, no mention is made of the tutor introducing the topic or stating any aims or expectations. Does this matter?

3.20(c) Now draw up a five-point 'recipe for successful learning' *from a student's perspective* based on your discussions about the above lesson sequence.

This sort of lesson format is probably familiar to you. It begins with the students' own experiences and broadens out by introducing new knowledge and challenging students to think about practical and finally abstract principles. This is one way of approaching learning. How else might the topic have been addressed? It could be argued that a good, informative, challenging lecture would have been as effective. What do you think? Your own lessons provide useful 'real life' case studies for reflection along these lines and will enable you to consider how effectively your students learn. Chapter 6, on assessment, will also introduce another dimension to the subject of effective learning.

Task 3.21

3.21(a) Consider in turn the following short 'pen sketches' of typical students. What barriers to learning might they encounter?

Julie is a 17-year-old who left secondary school a year ago with no qualifications. She has been unsuccessful in finding a suitable job although she has done some casual work in a fast-food restaurant. Julie is about to begin, somewhat reluctantly, a GNVQ Intermediate Course in Hospitality and Catering at her local FE college.

Steve is at the beginning of a three-year BA course in Media Studies and Sports Science at a 'new' university. He is 18 and has just left school with two A levels at grades C and D. Steve tried to get a job in leisure management, but has realized that he needs a degree if he is going to build a good career. His parents are unable to support him financially.

Mary is a 30-year-old mother of two, recently divorced. Her children are both of school age and she has now decided to do an Access course at her local FE college with a view to going on to HE. Mary left school at 16 with 4 O levels and did office work before her children were born.

Frank has recently retired at the age of 57. He left school at 14 and had been a shopkeeper all his life, working long hours. He now wants to keep his mind alert by joining a beginner's Spanish course at his local AE centre because he hopes to buy a holiday home in Spain.

3.21(b) Try to place the barriers you have identified into the categories of educational, institutional and societal. Do some of them overlap?

Some educational barriers might equally be considered to be institutional problems. For example, a Tourism tutor might be ill-equipped to help a student deal with a severe spelling problem. We might expect a learning support workshop to be available to give expert guidance and tuition. However, it *is* the responsibility of that Tourism tutor to ensure that the student is aware of the problem, to mark the student's work carefully and ensure that she or he gets whatever support is available. Many mature students lack confidence in their ability to learn, have low expectations of themselves or have memories of bad educational experiences. These, and other barriers to learning may have an educational aspect, but are intrinsically linked with institutional and particularly societal barriers.

Institutional barriers are sometimes harder to overcome. Any tutor who has fought to have a lift or even ramps installed to enable wheelchair access to parts of the building will know that while everyone agrees they are essential, the money is often slow in coming. The Association of University Teachers (AUT) in a summary of a piece of research into barriers to learning identified the following institutional barriers: poor quality of information; the high cost of many courses; the distance to travel; a confusing array of options; the time students have to give up to attend courses. This, they concluded, leads to a 'vicious spiral of unequal opportunities' (AUT 1997). The less people's potential is fulfilled, they observed, the less able and motivated they are to develop themselves.

The huge expansion in FE and HE in recent years has eroded some of the barriers to access that existed in the past. We have already mentioned the greater diversity of the post-16 student population. How have institutions fared in meeting the needs of such a wide range of students? Have new barriers to learning been created within institutions as a result?

This leads us into a discussion of the societal barriers to learning that people encounter, since education is a key part of social policy and is certainly the service which attracts the most attention and concern in the closing years of the twentieth century. The present government has expressed a firm commitment to 'lifelong learning' and a widening of access to education for all sections of society. Every study carried out prior to 1990 – for example the Further Education Unit's (FEU) survey *Marketing Adult and Continuing Education* (FEU 1987) – confirms that participation in PCE is predominantly composed of socio-economic groups A, B and C1. A study carried out by the National Institute of Adult and Continuing Education (NIACE) between 1987 and 1989 into the problem of non-participating groups in PCE (McGivney 1990) identified five distinct groups who were vastly under-represented. They were: unskilled/semi-skilled manual workers; unemployed people; women with dependent children; older adults (aged 50+); and ethnic minority groups. The study identified a wide range of reasons why people in these groups did not continue their education beyond school, some of which have already been mentioned. But the overarching barrier identified by all groups was that education was something that other people did and was perceived as not something they needed. How is the situation different now? Is it merely the case that more middle-class people are attending FE and HE? Has there been an attitudinal revolution among working-class people? Or is there now a more subtle coercive approach to including non-participatory groups through cuts in the benefit system? Have the 'ivory towers' been stormed or have the floodgates simply been opened?

Task 3.22

3.22(a) Consider what changes have taken place in either the FE, AE or HE sectors.

3.22(b) What barriers to learning have emerged or how has participation been widened and improved as a result of these changes?

3.22(c) How do *societal* barriers to learning link with *educational* and *institutional* barriers?

For whatever reason, participation is rising and ostensibly barriers are being removed and yet at the same time the recommendations of the recent Dearing Report on HE (Dearing 1997) to introduce tuition fees was warmly accepted by the Labour government and was due to be phased in in September 1998 together with the abolition of student grants. The aim is to encourage participation by people from poorer backgrounds while offsetting the burgeoning cost of HE by making the more well-off pay for their education. Does this move represent a democratizing of the HE system or will it restrict participation by people on average incomes still further?

This section has cast the net very widely over practical issues concerned with learning and has aimed to promote discussion about how we can ensure that our students achieve to the best of their ability and have high expectations of themselves. The next section seeks to explore the concept of learner autonomy.

3.5 *Learner autonomy*

KEY ISSUES

What distinguishes autonomous learner from learning autonomy?

Is learner autonomy concerned with the process of learning or is it an educational goal?

How do students develop good study skills?

If we brainstorm the variety of terms used to describe learning which is not teacher-centred, the list seems endless with little apparent distinction in the way labels are used. Tight (1996: 89) makes a distinction between what he calls 'learning concepts' which 'focus mainly on the perspective of the organisation providing education or training' and 'those which are more concerned with the perspective of the individual learner'. In the first category he places distance, flexible and open learning (which will be discussed in Chapter 5) as distinct from experiential, independent and self-directed learning where the shift from institutional responsibility to the individual leaves the learner in charge of and supposedly in control of their own learning.

The notion of the self-directed learner comes, as we have already seen, from the andragogical model of learning. While a variety of criticisms have been ranged at andragogy, nevertheless, many aspects have been incorporated into our understanding and practice in PCE. Not least, the self-directed, autonomous learner. Moore (1983: 163) suggests that:

> Autonomous learners – and this means most adults, most of the time – sometimes formally, often unconsciously, set objectives and define criteria for their achievement. Autonomous learners know, or find, where and how and from what human and other resources they may gather the information they require, collect ideas, practise skills and achieve their goals. They then judge the appropriateness of their new skills, information and ideas, eventually deciding whether their goals have been achieved or can be abandoned.

To what extent and to which groups of learners in PCE might this description fit? Perhaps not the average FE student, but what about groups in AE, or HE undergraduates? How many of the characteristics described by Moore do your learners display? Are our students 'naturally' self-directing, or is self-direction or learner autonomy something which the tutor can encourage through a particular style of teaching and which learners develop over a period of time? More importantly, should autonomy be more than knowing how to study and direct your learning? Can independent, critical thought be achieved autonomously? What are the implications for the role of the tutor?

It is increasingly the case that learners in all sectors of PCE need to develop their ability to study independently, to increase their 'learner autonomy'. Whatever the educational justifications that are made for 'learner autonomy', the reality is that cuts in course hours and the shift away from examination to project and assignment work means that students do spend much more time working alone or in groups without constant tutor guidance and supervision.

In FE, GNVQ is a good example of this. Moreover, independent study is now an integral part of all vocational courses and therefore the demands on both students and tutors are different from the tutor/student relationship associated with traditional craft courses. The 'autonomous learner' may seem to be an idealized description of many young people in FE and developing that autonomy is indeed a challenge for all concerned. This curriculum change is coupled with an explosion in the FE student population due to the collapse of the youth labour market and substantial budget cuts.

The shift in the AE curriculum towards more accredited courses puts more pressure on learners and tutors to achieve qualifications. In order to keep fees within affordable limits, course hours are often inadequate to cover all the syllabus adequately in class time. It is therefore essential that students engage in a significant amount of independent study.

In HE the shift is slightly different. Independent research and study has always been a defining feature of academic study and quite rightly so. In some respects the undergraduate epitomizes the autonomous learner described above. However, the recent massive expansion in HE has created several new problems. To begin with, the new expanded HE student population is much more diverse. There is now a greater proportion of mature people, part-time students, a higher social and ethnic mix and, arguably, a wider range of ability entering HE. Alongside this, the rise in student numbers has not been accompanied by a parallel increase in funding. Not surprisingly this has led to cuts in course hours and thus a much greater emphasis on independent study.

The possible reasons for these curriculum changes throughout PCE are discussed elsewhere, see Chapters 1 and 7 in particular. However, it is useful to consider how *you* would interpret 'learner autonomy' in your work and what emphasis you would place on it. Can real learner autonomy be achieved by the sorts of interpretations described above? The concept of 'autonomy' has taken on a new meaning in that it describes *how* learning takes place. What if, however, we define 'learner autonomy' as the achievement of intellectual freedom and critical thought through the mastery of a subject? Is this still an appropriate goal to aspire to? Can it be achieved through the *process* of 'autonomous learning', independent study, resource-based learning and workshops?

Task 3.23

Note down some of the arguments for and against autonomous learning.

In Section 3.4 we considered learner needs and the learning styles of our students. What often emerges from such analyses is that many students *do* require help and support in the way they approach learning. Learning how to learn is something that both students and tutors often ignore. We also considered effective learning in the classroom in Section 3.4. What we shall explore here are the skills that students need to enable them to learn and how they can be developed by the tutor. As teachers we routinely offer ad hoc guidance on how to approach a piece of work, or perhaps we have a 'study skills' handout that we give to each student with advice on time management and approaches to reading and so on. Some courses begin with a study skills module covering much the same ground. The essential point about study skills or learning to learn is that it must be done in *context*; it must be applied to the subject to be studied.

Task 3.24

3.24(a) Choose one of your typical teaching sessions and write down the sequence of activities in the lesson. Organize the information in three columns. In the first column write down what *you* do throughout the lesson; in the second column record the parallel student activity. When you have done that, look at each student activity and identify what learning strategies your students need at each stage. For example:

- Teacher activity strategy: introductory talk.
- Student activity: listen, take notes.
- Learning: assimilate information, extract key points and write them down.

3.24(b) Now examine the learning strategies you have identified. Are all your students able to apply these strategies effectively? Which ones could you give help with during the lesson? Which ones require a longer-term plan to develop? How can you facilitate and support this?

Whatever subject you are teaching, students need to develop effective study skills. It is essential that learning strategies are acquired and practised in the classroom if students are going to be able to learn effectively on their own.

The diversity of learners in the post-compulsory sector of education is as wide as the types of courses and programmes on which they enrol. Faced with such diversity, and the pressures on tutors to respond to every individual's learning needs, it is not surprising that we sometimes lose sight of the similarities between learners and their common goals. This chapter has introduced a variety of aspects of learning and has sought to relate theoretical perspectives to contemporary issues and professional practice.

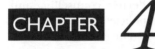

TEACHING AND THE MANAGEMENT OF LEARNING

4.1 What is Chapter 4 about?

We have already considered the teacher's role in the learning process in Chapter 3. In this chapter we focus on the teacher as manager of the learning environment and the skills and knowledge which we require in order to carry out this duty as competently as possible. Teacher skills will be looked at again in Chapter 7, where there will be a discussion of planning as a curriculum process and a teaching skill. In Chapter 5 we examine the incorporation of effective resources in the learning process, which is another facet of the teacher's role.

No teaching takes place in a vacuum. Even though we may see teaching as a partly planned and partly spontaneous act, our approach to it, our interpretation of our role, our attitude to our students and our view of what we should be teaching are shaped by a variety of factors. These include our personal belief system, our own experience of being taught, our personality and our theoretical understanding of the teaching and learning process.

In Section 4.2 we will look at varying approaches to teaching, along a continuum from didactic to learner-centred. Section 4.3 will focus on the management of learning groups, reviewing the characteristics of different groups of learners, as already discussed in Chapter 3, and moving on to an exploration of group culture, structure, effectiveness and management techniques. Section 4.4 considers the practical management skills which are needed when dealing with groups with challenging behaviour. Rule-making related to deviance, labelling and stereotyping will also be examined. The role of the tutor is considered in Section 4.5, with an emphasis on the skills which are necessary for effective counselling and guidance, a consideration of equal opportunities policies relating to race, gender and perceived ability, and a comment on current legislation on these issues. In the final section we look at the teacher as manager of the learning environment, consider a range of settings to maximize effective learning and look at legal aspects of health and safety policies.

4.2 *Approaches to teaching*

KEY ISSUES

What are the various approaches to teaching?

What are the origins of these approaches?

Which of them are appropriate for us?

How do these approaches relate to strategies?

'Teachers do have theories and belief systems that influence their perceptions, plans and actions' (Calderhead 1987: 107).

Our approach to teaching is a highly complex process, which requires us to understand theories of learning, our ideological view of our role as a teacher, our particular learning context, our subject, the environment and the background and expectations of our students. Various labels are often used to describe these approaches such as 'auto-didactic' or 'facilitative'. Broadly speaking, our approach will depend on our beliefs about our role and that of our learners at a given period in our professional career. If we adopt the view that the mere act of teaching is for us a learning process then our beliefs may change and our approach may modify. Our approach at the start of our professional life, during training, is modelled largely on a combination of our own prior learning experiences and theoretical representations of the craft of teaching. Gradually we add to these the following: increased classroom practice where trial and error are so crucial; an awareness of and exposure to psychological factors governing student attitude and attainment; and the ongoing reflection which reshapes our view of what we are doing, and consequently causes us to revise our practice.

Our personal approach to teaching is a unique one which combines all the factors we have mentioned so far with the individual stamp of our personality. At any given point in time we may find ourselves using a variety of approaches which lie along a continuum from didactic to learner-centred. Minton (1991) develops these these views with a matrix, shown in Figure 4.1.

Figure 4.1 Minton's matrix of control

Teacher control		Lecture
		Demonstration
		Discussion (structured)
	Less control	Discussion (unstructured)
		Seminar
		Tutorial
	Shared control	Practical
		Simulation and games
		Role-play
		Resource-based learning
		Films/TV programmes
		Visits
	Student control	Distance learning/flexistudy
		Discovery projects/research
Least control		Real-life experience

Source: Minton 1991: 112.

Task 4.1

In pairs discuss how the content/process-oriented continuum influences how you teach. What strategies do you regularly use? List them.

Task 4.2

Decide in pairs where the following strategies might lie along this continuum: demonstrations, negotiating own line of enquiry, peer group teaching, questioning.

Rogers (1996) finds four categories of teaching methods: presentation methods (teacher activities such as demonstration, exposition, use of blackboard, text or audio-visual media); participatory methods (interaction between teacher and learner, or learner and learner, through for example, questions, discussion, small or large group work); discovery methods (in which the learners on their own or in groups work on tasks, exploring or discovering knowledge for themselves through practice, experiments, reading and writ-ing); evaluatory methods (in which tests, quizzes and role-plays become the means for further learning).

Task 4.3

Consider the following subjects and decide in small groups on the balance of presentation, participatory and discovery methods which might be used in planning: pottery, mathematics, a foreign language, car mechanics, food hygiene, basic literacy skills.

What then is the origin of these various approaches? Our approach to teaching is usually based on a theory of teaching and the teacher's role, which is part of a curriculum ideology. So Meighan (quoted in Preedy 1989: 42), states that a theory of teaching is one of the following components which curriculum planners must address: 'a theory of teaching and the teacher's role, formal or informal, authoritarian or democratic, an interest in outcomes or processes, narrow or wide'. Morrison and Ridley (Preedy 1989: 46–7) expand Meighan's components of ideology into a consideration of how a teacher's role might be determined by a particular view of the world, categorizing these ideologies according to three emphases: knowledge (classical humanism, liberal humanism, traditionalism, academicism and conservatism); society (instrumentalism, revisionism, economic renewal, reconstructionism, and democratic socialism); and the individual (progressivism, child-centredness and romanticism). (For further discussion see Preedy 1989, Ch. 4.) Morrison and Ridley's analysis is useful in helping us to reflect on our own ideological position and to identify the dominant ideologies which characterize the contexts in which we operate. We may, for example, decide that our own views conflict with those of our colleagues, our department, the institutions we work for or national policies.

Task 4.4

Educational policies are established according to certain sets of beliefs or ideologies. In groups, discuss the dominant ideologies inherent in current educational policies in Britain with which you are familiar.

Awareness of the origin of approaches helps us to understand the strategies we employ. Strategies are the practical application of approaches. In practice we often use a variety of approaches, which are influenced by a number of factors:

- our understanding of their purpose in the fulfilment of the learning goals;
- our relationship with the group;
- consideration of resources, time and equipment;
- balance, variety and maintenance of student interest;
- our breadth of experience and willingness to experiment.

Task 4.5

On your own, choose a sequence of three lessons you have recently taught with the same group. Which strategies did you use and why? If you were to repeat the same sequence of lessons would you include/preclude other strategies?

Each of the factors listed above can be broken down into further components. For example, under the umbrella heading of 'our relationship with the group' we need to think about:

- how long we have worked with the group;
- the profile of adults as learners, i.e. prior learning experience;
- how cooperative the group is;
- the attitudes of members of the group to participatory activities;
- the age of the learners – young or older adults.

We can test the effectiveness of various approaches through the processes of assessment and evaluation. These will be discussed in greater depth in Chapter 6. Informal and formal assessment methods can provide us with indications of the success, economy and enjoyment of adopting various approaches.

Finally, there is need for flexibility in approach. In the teaching process we need to be prepared to experiment and accept that sometimes strategies do not work with certain groups. We need also to be alert to economy. There is often tension between process and product, in the sense that time constraints may dictate the use of more formal methods of instruction. The age of our learners means that if we are using what are perceived to be 'new' teaching methods, such as role-play or group work, we may need to justify these methods to help participants learn more effectively. We need to be able to respond to changes which may be imposed upon us and yet argue a case for the methods that we find to be effective.

4.3 *Management of learning groups*

KEY ISSUES

What are the major classroom management techniques?

Management of a variety of learning groups: formation, development, culture

In considering the management of learning groups we presuppose a duty to make learning, both as an individual and a group experience, as rich and beneficial as possible for all within that group. So it is important for us to consider various techniques of group management. When we talk of classroom management in the primary and secondary sectors we talk very often in terms of control. This would seem somewhat inappropriate in relation to adults, particularly those who are classified as 'mature'.

In our management capacity, therefore, it is important for us to appreciate how groups function, the stages they go through, the processes which characterize learning groups and the way in which individuals in a group assume roles and tasks. We need to consider the conditions under which a healthy group culture emerges and understand our role in this.

In this section we will look at group culture, group structure and group effectiveness. Awareness of how groups function can be beneficial to the teacher in building self-esteem, developing a positive feeling towards the group and understanding some of the difficulties which characterize most groups.

We can define group culture as the essence of a group which makes it unique. Each learning group we have ever belonged to has in some way been different, and many of us are familiar with 'parallel' learning groups, i.e. groups working towards identical educational objectives and yet which function very differently and which, significantly, affect our perceptions of ourselves as tutors and the group as learners. It is common to hear tutors discuss groups in terms of liking and disliking, having a good or bad 'feel', being cooperative or the opposite. Sometimes the discussion changes focus, so that particular individuals within the group are cited, sometimes as assuming a role within the group which particularly affects its make-up. It is probably true to say that often our discussions go no further, that we do not probe the behaviour of particular individuals. We may also be hesitant or reluctant to analyse our own role within the group, perhaps out of a mixture of fear, indifference or laziness. Such analysis is important nonetheless. We may spend a lot of time planning our classes, formulating sound learning objectives and providing interesting resources, but if our groups are problematic then effective learning will not take place. We need to appreciate how groups function.

Task 4.6

Think of a learning group you are or have been part of. What is the group experience like? Do/did you enjoy the group? Is/was there a sense of cooperation? Do/did members of the group enjoy learning with each other? Work in small groups.

The group culture is created by the interaction and interdependence between the members, and the feelings, beliefs, attitudes and personalities which they bring to the group at a given time. Theorists such as Freire and Rogers, as interpreted by Jarvis (1995), inform us that learning is an 'emancipatory experience which may involve a change in self organisation and perception' and that 'much socially useful learning is learning the process of learning and retaining an openness to experience, so that the process of change may be incorporated into the self' (p. 99). If we accept this view it follows that the group is not a static entity, that it will be continually reshaping itself according to the way in which its individual members are responding to their learning environment. It is little wonder that we sometimes find group behaviour mercurial and unpredictable, and that on occasions the experience of trying to lead or manage a group can be difficult, bewildering and exhausting. Rogers (1983: 148) notes the following features which stem from teaching adults in groups: they provide a supportive environment for learning; a constant challenge to the learner; resources to build richer and more complex structures for learning; and they have a life of their own, which can assist the learning.

It is also useful for tutors to take note of Rogers' stress on group autonomy and recognize that the group does have a life of its own which is distinct from the tutor. It is interesting to observe the difference in the way in which a group behaves when a tutor absents themselves for a period of time. Such observation can tell us much about the tutor's role in and importance to the group, whether it is that of a facilitator or controller. A further reinforcement of the notion that a group has its own life is the consideration of two or more tutors sharing the teaching of a group and making comparisons. This can lead to challenging thoughts on self-perception and our perception of others.

Individual group members will assume roles which will be determined by a plethora of factors: our previous experience of being part of a group; our particular needs and stage of intellectual growth at the time of forming part of the group; our personality (whether we are introvert or extrovert, for example); our assumptions about how a group should function; and what constitutes acceptable and unacceptable behaviour and our belief about others.

As a group becomes familiar its members may shed old roles and assume new ones. This can create tension and conflict but has the function of ensuring that the group remains shifting and dynamic. Here are some of the roles which people play in groups: facilitator, passive aggressor, questioner, distractor, joker, withdrawer, aggressor, monopolizer, rescuer, harmonizer, leader, complainer, projector, the nice guy.

Task 4.7

Individually, think of a current or recent teaching group. Do you recognize the roles listed above and can you add to the list? What is your understanding of the terms?

When a group member plays the same role consistently a pattern of behaviour emerges. This is distinct from infrequent displays of passive and entire groups with challenging behaviour. We will start with cases of individuals whom we find difficult.

Our response to behaviour which we find irritating, disturbing or destructive can vary considerably according to our personal view and experience of the kind of behaviour which is acceptable in the classroom. It will also depend on our personal levels of tolerance in general and on our mood on a particular day! As teachers, we tend with experience to establish a set of personal rules which set boundaries to our acceptance of student behaviour. However, we are not always good at communicating these rules, perhaps because we associate this process with working with children, where the importance of establishing classroom rules is a matter of course. Thus it can take adults longer to work out our rules, often to the point where they unknowingly break them, and it is only then that we spell them out!

As with children, consistency of approach is important, as is fairness to all. As mentioned at the end of Section 4.4, our message needs to be that it is the behaviour which is unacceptable, not the person.

We may need to learn to be more tolerant, but we do need to know our own boundaries if we are to send out consistent messages. We should also recognize that our response to behaviour can be the result of our own 'baggage', which explains individual differences in attitude.

Task 4.9

In pairs, specify ten rules which form a consistent part of your classroom practice, e.g. 'students are expected to be punctual'. Compare your lists with other colleagues.

Task 4.10

Here is a list of behaviours which can cause irritation. Rank them in order of how you think they might affect you:

- talking at the same time as you;
- exchanging glances which imply criticism;
- students doing their own work in your class time;
- interrupting;
- sullenness;
- refusal to cooperate in activities;
- excessive joking;
- sarcasm;
- fidgeting;
- whispering;
- challenging.

Now discuss the underlying cause of such behaviour and relate this to the attitude of the learner and what she or he might be trying to tell the tutor, even if not in the most direct way.

Faced with a range of examples of unwanted behaviour we need to look at practical strategies for dealing with it, including self-talk. Self-talk can be a positive or negative force in such circumstances. Sometimes, when we realize that a person's behaviour is adversely affecting us and the rest of the group we begin to engage in disabling self-talk of the 'I can't deal with this' variety. It is important to recognize this as disabling and steer ourselves along a more positive avenue of self-talk, which will give us patience and calmness and enable us to maintain control over our feelings. Here are examples of underlying beliefs which we may bring into the classroom which may be barriers to managing difficult behaviour: being liked ('I must always be liked and valued by significant people in my life'); being competent ('I must be seen to be competent in all situations'); having my own way ('I must always have my own way in a class and my plans must always work out') (adapted from Egan 1994: 18).

Faced with a situation which threatens to undermine any of these tenets it is easy for us to allow disabling self-talk to prevent us from responding positively. Examining such beliefs can be challenging, even painful, but may reveal useful insights into our view of ourselves as a teacher. You may wish to reflect individually on them.

What our internal dialogues need to be about is identifying behaviour, telling ourselves that we *can* often do something positive, that we are probably being supported by some others in the group and that the behaviour is not being directed personally at us as individuals. We need to deal quickly and firmly with unwanted behaviour, but with humour and tact. Our body language is crucial in helping us to stay calm. Sarcasm, or making a person look foolish can be temporarily effective, but are undesirable and of course do not address the underlying cause of the problem. They are natural but ill-advised solutions.

Task 4.11

Think of a difficulty you encountered and relate it to a colleague. Role-play the situation and through the role-play explore the behaviour, as well as possible methods of dealing with it.

Labelling theory is used to explain the concept of deviance, which arises when a person or group applies a judgement to a person who is perceived to break social rules. Of course, a set of rules for one group may be quite different for another. There may also be a variation from culture to culture. There are many dangers inherent in labelling, for example: it affects self-esteem and self-advocacy; it may restrict learning potential; a label tends to stick to a person for a long time; it limits one's perception of the person being labelled; there is a tendency to conform to the characteristics suggested by the label.

Task 4.12

It is at this point that we should stop to consider the types of label with which we might come into contact. Examples might be 'troublemaker', 'thick', 'lazy', 'manic'. Some labels are overtly damning, others less so. Make a list of labels with which you are familiar.

Self-labelling based on previous learning experience can be a powerful barrier to learning and can be used as an excuse or defence mechanism. This requires us to challenge the very idea of labels as well as the role they tell us we should play. In other words, we must discourage students from taking refuge in their labels, which might prevent them from shedding them, although this can be a difficult process.

We can define stereotyping as the desire to categorize a person or people too simplistically, so that we have a fixed, conventionalized representation of them. The effect of this process is to strip them of individuality and 'fix' them into a role beyond the parameters of which we do not regard them. Thus we can see the link between stereotyping and labelling. Stereotyping according to gender and race is very prevalent in society today, despite the increase in equal opportunities policies. We need therefore to exercise vigilance in all aspects of our teaching in order to ensure that we do not reinforce stereotypes. If we take gender as an issue, this will involve ensuring that we distribute learning tasks without discrimination, and that our resources do not reflect stereotypical views of traditional roles which men and women take, even at the most subliminal level. Role-play can be a useful method of exploring such issues and developing empathetic responses. With younger adults it is important to consider that we may be the only person in their lives who is prepared to challenge stereotypical views, since very young adults in particular are still influenced in their prejudices by their peers and the media.

Task 4.13

With a partner, think of examples of xenophobia which you have witnessed in your classes. Think of activities you could do with classes to address these issues.

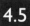 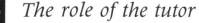

4.5 *The role of the tutor*

KEY ISSUES

The need to be flexible is a key part of the teacher's role

The role of the tutor varies in and out of a formal classroom setting

Teacher skills in counselling and guidance are central to student learning

Teachers have an important role in promoting equal opportunities

We have looked so far in this chapter at strategies for managing groups of learners in terms of selecting appropriate teaching strategies and understanding how learners behave within groups. Our focus in this section is on the role of the tutor, which, as Walklin (1990) tells us is multi-faceted. We will look at the following areas: flexibility; counselling and guidance; and equal opportunities.

Flexibility

The tutor's responsibility in ensuring the effective delivery of the curriculum through preparation and efficient management of learning is overlaid with the all-important dimension of flexibility. The need to be flexible is determined by the fact that every individual teaching group we have ever encountered is unique and it therefore follows that our role and style of leadership within each group is unique. Since roles of group members are interdependent (Lovell 1980: 163) the very act of having to negotiate our role within each different learning group reinforces our experience of flexibility. Flexibility is also a prerequisite to working within an education system such as we have in Britain, which can be stressful. Our world consists of meeting deadlines, working irregular and or unsocial hours, juggling teaching and administrative responsibilities and dealing with the unpredictable.

Task 4.14

Choose a typical day in your teaching week and talk through it with a colleague. What might be the unpredictable elements?

The challenge for us as tutors is to achieve a balance. This consists of being flexible about our expectations of our students, and yet demonstrating stability in the following: efficient organization of the learning environment; consistency; and the ability to establish codes of conduct. In other words, we need to be flexible, but from a stable base. This involves thinking through areas of our teaching where we are prepared to entertain flexibility and those where we are not.

Task 4.15

In small groups discuss the following areas and decide which require greater or lesser degrees of flexibility: assignment deadlines; punctuality; class times; leaving the class early; responding to requests about modes of delivery. Try to relate to any experience you have had so far and also consider whether you feel that the age of the learners has any bearing on your thoughts.

A further tension which we need to consider involves our dealings with individuals within the group. Do we show the same degree of flexibility towards each individual? Are we consistent generally in our behaviour with the group? Any inconsistency on our part in this respect may lead to negative feelings on the part of individuals who perceive themselves as being treated unfairly. We are setting up a 'barrier to equality' (Reece and Walker 1994), an issue which we will pick up later in this section.

We need to be flexible in delivery and approach and recognize that approaches which are successful with some groups are not appropriate for others, and to this end we should be prepared to be flexible through experimenting with our activities and approaches in order to best achieve our objectives and learning outcomes. We also need to consider our response to individuals. Students will at various times need to make special requests, to be treated in some way differently from others in the group. We need in these situations to exercise discretion and fairness, ensuring that our decisions are fair to all. It can often be useful to engage the support and advice of a colleague or line manager when making awkward decisions.

Our role within the group is a further area where flexibility is crucial. There are many roles which we might have in our teaching groups. Here are some which Walklin (1990: 246) has established: change agent and innovator; communicator; counsellor and coach; helper and supporter; implementer; monitor and evaluator; motivator and team leader; needs identifier and adviser; organizer and planner; staff developer; teaching and learning media expert. Clearly in our groups we may find ourselves playing several of these roles.

Task 4.16

As a personal reflection activity, make a list of the roles which you play in two teaching groups.

It is important to point out that we cannot successfully play all these roles and we need to take account of ourselves as individuals in deciding what exactly is appropriate for us to take on.

Counselling and guidance

Egan (1994: 18) states:

> research on human problem solving would have been more profitable had it attempted to incorporate ideas from learning theory. Even more so, research on learning would have borne more fruit had Thorndike not cast out problem solving. This lack of synergy has limited the contributions of these two paradigms to the helping professions.

An understanding of counselling skills is important for a tutor in enhancing the learning process. These skills can help us lead students towards an appreciation of barriers to learning they may be experiencing. Counselling skills can also help students to establish personal targets and goals in order to manage their learning more effectively and build or develop self-esteem and self-awareness. Counselling as a tutor is an integral part of facilitating student learning and involves an understanding of motivation, self-esteem and learner autonomy (see Chapter 3).

Some counselling skills are so familiar to us that we perceive them as being teaching skills and not part of the counselling process: listening, advising and clarifying are obvious examples. Some of our classroom activities also reflect techniques used in counselling such as brainstorming, which Egan (1994: 229) describes as a 'tool for divergent thinking'. Problem-solving activities which we set our students can be used to help them become better learners.

Reece and Walker (1994: 130) list the following counselling skills as being of use to teachers: ice breaking, listening, clarifying, reflecting back, summarizing, advising and target setting.

Task 4.17

Think of a teaching situation in the last week. How many of the skills listed above have you used? Are there any other skills you have used?

There are other communication skills which may be less familiar. They include: attending skills; active listening (being attentive to verbal and non-verbal messages); empathy; and probing. Attending skills, empathy and probing are essential communication skills in that they help us to try to understand exactly what students are saying to us, when sometimes

OFL is not new. It has been around in some form for quite a time, although without many of the features we believe are important to its success today. Most people have heard of correspondence courses and the Open University even if they have not had direct experience of them. It is these initiatives that are the forerunners to today's systems of OFL. Increasingly, OFL is being linked to the development of CBL and the use of electronic communication such as email and teleconferencing. However, OFL as an approach to assisting learning is a concept that would exist regardless of the technology used to deliver it.

We are focusing on OFL in this part of the chapter for two reasons:

1 OFL appears to be 'taking off' within many post-compulsory establishments. Many colleges for example are now investing in open learning centres. No doubt they see this partly as a sound economic development but they may also sense a growing popularity for this type of approach among individual students and businesses approaching colleges for training.
2 OFL is very dependent on good quality resources. The choice and design of these resources play a vital part in helping students achieve their learning objectives. Part of this section will be devoted to the preparation of 'conventional' open learning materials. We have looked elsewhere at some aspects of IT-based approaches.

You will encounter a variety of terms in the literature of learning resources including distance learning and 'flexistudy', which quite often mean the same thing or at least share many attributes. However, 'open learning' is a term generally used to describe courses flexibly designed to meet individual requirements. It follows that open learning systems try to remove barriers that prevent attendance on more traditional courses and therefore usually include arrangements for people to learn at the time, place and pace that suits their circumstances. Restrictions placed on students are under constant review in open learning systems. Another key characteristic of open learning is its student focus. There is often an emphasis on learner choice, on negotiation of outcomes, on student self-assessment and on learner evaluation of the modules. Materials are designed to suit the learner. Finally, most open learning systems require specially prepared or adapted materials with which students can interact. There should be a variety of resources available for use in different ways. OFL is not, however, 'old-fashioned' distance learning, and appropriate tutorial support and the use of support groups are important elements in any OFL arrangements. In this sense the mode of tutorial support (e.g. 'face-to-face' or email) is largely unimportant: it is the quality and effectiveness of this support which really counts.

It is not difficult to see why OFL is growing rapidly: busy adults prefer flexible arrangements which fit round their lives; they like to work at their own pace (without being embarrassed); they like access to tutorial support, but are less keen on teachers 'leaning over their shoulders' all the time. OFL can give learners ownership of the process through the ability to negotiate how learning is achieved. It can allow students to gain confidence by working through a course in manageable chunks achieving success at each step. OFL can make it easy to revisit the 'difficult bits' whenever necessary. Businesses have also been quick to see the benefits of this approach to training. It causes less disruption of work schedules, training resources are better used, and after initial 'tooling up costs' it can be a relatively cheap option for developing some skills, freeing resources to be spent in other areas. OFL can target specific training needs as employees can tackle only those modules that are needed; they don't have to sit through an entire taught course. Many large enterprises like Ford and British Airways use OFL extensively. They are attracted by the best schemes which use a range of very sophisticated technologies to put over information in a way that speeds understanding and helps retention.

For colleges and training centres the advantages are various. The institution may attract more students and therefore much-needed cash, and OFL has been used to reduce programme costs in some college courses. Some lecturers are attracted to it because it is learner-centred, and enables them to adopt a number of different support roles.

Task 5.11

It has been suggested that elements of one of the courses you teach could be redesigned as open learning modules. Students would be expected to use self-study packages, work at their own pace, and use a range of resources. Tutorial support would be available, but not necessarily from you! Choose one of the courses you teach and consider the following:

5.11(a) Which elements might it be possible to deliver through open learning modules? Why have you chosen these elements as the most appropriate for open learning?

5.11(b) What would be the major advantages and disadvantages of using open learning for parts of the course you have chosen?

5.11(c) In order for open learning to be successfully integrated into your course, what organizational elements would need to change in your establishment (e.g. timetabling)? What training would you and your colleagues need to enhance your skills and to enable you to support open learning most effectively?

The best OFL schemes use high quality, carefully designed resources such as interactive video, access to online databases, audio tapes, articles and study guides. Such resources are expensive because they take time to prepare. There are numerous problems facing anyone trying to design open learning materials, as well as problems facing those trying to use them! The materials tend to be 'one-way'. You do not get the instant feedback of the classroom where, if a topic is difficult or your approach ineffective, learners will soon let you know one way or another. Therefore, great care has to be taken when choosing or preparing resources for open learners and when writing the instructions or guides that tell the learners how to use the resource.

For example, when preparing open learning materials for your students or when using commercially produced resources, you need to know your students' characteristics as independent learners. What is their reading level for example? If you write in too abstract, technical or complex a manner, they might be easily lost but if you simplify your language too much they may feel patronized! Also factors such as motivation, peer group support and study skills are important to consider in this respect.

In the classroom you can provide many different forms of support for your students: arousing interest through enthusiastic delivery, and linking ideas to students' interests; clarifying objectives and their relevance to the students; presenting difficult concepts or skills in a number of different ways; providing opportunities for practice and giving immediate feedback. Can open learning materials be a satisfactory, if not perfect, substitute?

Open learning materials cannot be written like an ordinary textbook. Textbooks focus on content and not support or guidance. Textbooks are usually organized according to the logic of the subject rather than the logic of learning. They take the perspective of the subject specialist rather than that of the learner. They require the physical presence and support of a teacher. Open learning materials are more complex in structure and function.

Task 5.12

Do this activity with a colleague if you can. You might choose a resource that you both use.

5.12(a) Select a written learning resource currently in use on one of your courses. It may be an instruction booklet, an introduction to a topic, a written briefing for a task or assignment, a list of legal definitions etc.

5.12(b) Examine your chosen material for readability, clarity, layout and tone.

5.12(c) Comment briefly on how you would improve the chosen resource to enhance communication with the learner.

Staff who are integrating open learning into their courses often want to use existing materials and packages such as standard textbooks, videos and computer programs. They do not want to design and produce all their own resources. The solution is to write a study guide to supplement the existing materials, to compensate for any weaknesses those materials might have and to guide the learner through the resources.

A study guide might include any or all the following features (adapted from Powell 1991: 45–8):

- Your overviews and/or summaries of the topic.
- Concept maps or other diagrams showing how the main topics and ideas are related.
- Learning objectives.
- An annotated bibliography.
- Guidance as to which chapters/sections to study and which to ignore.
- Specially-written (or audiotaped) alternative explanations, to be studied instead of sections in the material that you think are inaccurate, biased, out of date or confusing.
- Local examples or case studies which you have prepared because they will be more appealing than those (if any) in the existing material.
- Your paragraph-by-paragraph commentary on the argument expressed in the text.
- Questions and activities based on the material, section by section.
- Model or specimen answers to activities, and/or checklists whereby learners can evaluate their own responses to questions or activities that seem likely to produce unpredictable responses.
- Suggestions for practical work or experimental activity (e.g. guidelines or worksheets).
- A glossary of technical terms.
- A self-assessed test related to the objectives.
- Questions to discuss with fellow learners.
- Instructions for an assignment to be sent to a tutor for comment and/ or marking.

The role of the library resource centre in supporting learning

Inspection reports and research into the use of libraries have drawn attention to a valuable, and very expensive learning resource frequently underused and undervalued. In the past the library has often been seen as a 'warehouse' for books and of marginal relevance to many of the practical subjects taught in PCE. This has recently been changing. The growth of OFL, more assignment-driven courses, assessment criteria that include research skills and processing information, and an increase in the number of part-time adult learners who want to do independent work have brought radical changes to the 'old college library', turning it, in many cases, into a learning resource centre.

In such centres, the range of resources available is obviously important but the atmosphere, the provision of spaces for different types of work, and the skills support available are equally important.

> **Task 5.13**
>
> 5.13(a) What role(s) does the library resource centre play in your institution?
>
> 5.13(b) How important is your library resource centre in the development of your students' skills and abilities? Would your students' learning suffer if you didn't have a learning resource centre? How?
>
> 5.13(c) What changes would you like to see to the learning resource centre in your institution to make it a better support to learning? Think broadly: for example, range of resources, layout, staffing, access etc.

Development of student skills in using learning resources

It is a cliché to say that students now have access to more information and a wider range of resources than ever before. The question is, can they make effective use of these resources?

This question has become more pressing in recent years because of the changing patterns in PCE. Many courses, for example those approved by Edexcel, require students to tackle complex assignments needing a lot of research. Open learning is very resource-based and poses enormous problems for students without information-handling skills. Many adult learners have not studied for years and find the battery of resources facing them very daunting. Many professions (such as policing and nursing) now require critical reflection as part of their training. The responsibility is much more on students to carry out their own independent study and research. Without adequate skills, students learn ineffectively and increase their chances of failure. To help students become effective and successful learners and achieve their potential, teachers need to consider the following.

What study skills do students need to possess in order to get through the courses they follow and to cope with the work they are set? For example, do they need to be able to take notes, to extract information from written and visual sources? To synthesize information from different sources? Can they formulate good questions? Can they analyse data and generate hypotheses? (These skills apply to the use of IT as well as to printed resources.) Student-centred learning and independent learning can place enormous pressures on students, highlighting any problems that they have studying and dealing with information.

Who should develop these skills? Many lecturers believe that students should have developed key skills by the time they get to college or training school. They feel that there is no time to spend on general study skills in an overcrowded course. Help and support is usually available to those students who conspicuously lack certain skills, e.g. literacy (as a form of 'crisis management'), but what about those students who struggle through assignments, learning very inefficiently but passing? Should they go to special skills workshops or should skills work be provided as an integral part of their subject courses?

How can these skills be developed? Research has shown that there are some clear principles underpinning the development of these key skills:

- Relevance is crucial. Skills are developed using realistic and purposeful tasks, not little 'made-up' exercises. Skills need to be 'built into' coursework, but not buried in it. Skill development doesn't take place where skills are invisible to the students using them which leads on to the next point.
- Students need to use their skills, to reflect on what they have done and then to try out improved strategies. Students react badly to being told the 'right way' to take notes, write essays etc. They need support as they examine their existing study skills and strategies and work out how to make them more effective.
- Effective use of study skills needs to be valued in assessment and direct feedback on the use of such skills should be given to students.
- A variety of teaching approaches is needed to suit different styles of learning.

When considering resources to promote effective learning, the question of students' abilities to use the resources must surely be a central issue.

The notions of OFL, 'distance learning' and RBL can easily become confused and even treated as aspects of the 'same thing'. However, RBL is a term most properly restricted to, in the words of Gibbs and Parsons (1994), 'the use of mainly printed materials, written, collated or signposted by tutors, as a substitute for some aspects of teaching and library use . . . The focus is on full-time students, learning "on campus" but more independently through the use of print-based learning resources.' It does not follow however that these resources need necessarily be accessed by students in the conventional manner: they can just as easily be provided to students, for example, using the organization's own computer network.

Developing RBL

Rather than trying to introduce a full-blown RBL approach immediately think instead of working more gradually towards RBL. Gibbs and Parsons (1994: 31) suggest the following:

- finding out what resources are already available for one topic on one of your programs;
- starting to collect resource materials around topics, cataloguing them and producing resource packs;
- collecting handouts and programs information together into a program guide;
- using an existing resource, possibly one produced elsewhere or commercially, for one week or for one topic instead of your usual teaching;

- attempting to write a learning resource yourself for the use of your students for a single topic on a program that is usually taught conventionally;
- starting to replace selected taught sessions by word processing your notes together with a guide to activities and other resources associated with these notes;
- creating a 'reader' (a collection of reading materials, usually extracts from non-book sources – be aware of copyright considerations) for one part of your program;
- finding others, either within your own organization or elsewhere, with whom to write material;
- Looking for funding (e.g. through sponsorship) to support the development and costs of production of more RBL materials.

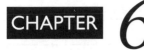

6 ASSESSMENT

6.1 What is Chapter 6 about?

The formal and informal assessment of students is becoming a large part of the work of teachers throughout PCE. Although external awarding bodies may offer guidance and training with respect to assessment, and assessor awards aim to equip tutors with the ability to assess students taking a wider range of qualifications (see Section 6.5), it is the responsibility of tutors in their classrooms to assess and monitor student progress. This chapter aims to provide a basis for developing tutors' expertise in creating and using the range of assessment strategies necessary to do this.

Section 6.2 looks at our experience of being assessed, both inside and outside an educational context, emphasizing the significance of key events both to ourselves and our students. Our negative experiences could have resulted from errors in the construction and use of the assessment concerned and there will be a consideration of the concepts of validity and reliability and the role they play in the structure and use of assessment. Crucial too is the type of referencing used and its relation to the aims and objectives of learning, and this is considered in Section 6.3. Section 6.4 will examine a range of assessment techniques and their suitability for particular learning strategies, while Section 6.5 looks particularly at the elements of competence-based assessment and provides guidance and support for those engaged in assessor awards. Finally, if assessment is to be of any enduring value in the learning process, it must be appropriately recorded and reported and Section 6.6 considers how most effectively the reviewing of student progress can be achieved.

6.2 *Assessment: ourselves and our students*

KEY ISSUES

How might assessment affect teachers and learners?

Why do we assess?

How might we improve the quality of assessment?

Just as many of us, consciously or unconsciously, tend to use those teaching strategies we experienced as learners, so our own experience of being assessed plays a key role in the development of our repertoire as a teacher.

Task 6.1: Our own experience

6.1(a) Consider the experiences you've had of being assessed, either in an educational setting, such as the 11+, GCSE, A level or vocational exam, or outside, such as scout or guide badges, life saving-awards or job interviews. Choose one example of assessment which had a positive effect and one which had a negative effect.

6.1(b) Share these with the group. Are there particular features common to the group regarding what was positive or negative in their experiences?

At the risk of stating the obvious, assessment which had a positive effect on you was more likely to be that which you were successful at! But, quite apart from the high quality of your performance, this could have been because you were aware of what was required or that the assessment itself was a fair test of your learning. Conversely, negative experiences could have been the result of misunderstanding the nature of the assessment or not having any feedback on your performance. Figure 6.1 presents a list of remarks made by a range of students in post-compulsory settings about the assessment of their work.

Task 6.2: Assessing your students

6.2(a) Repeat Task 6.1 only this time choose three examples of assessment you have recently completed with your students. How do you think they felt about these experiences?

6.2(b) Share your views with the rest of the group.

Figure 6.1 Reactions to assessment

'When we have a test, I forget everything straight afterwards.'

'Our teacher takes so long to mark our work, we've forgotten what it was about by the time we get it back.'

'I'd like more constructive criticism from our art tutor. She just says "Great" all the time. When I challenge her, she claims she doesn't want to be too prescriptive.'

'I was delighted to get 85 per cent for my last essay . . . until I discovered everyone in the group got between 85 and 95 per cent.'

'Our lecturer only points out what you get wrong at the bottom of a piece of work . . . never how you could have got it right.'

'My mate's dad does all his assignments. My mate just word-processes them. It doesn't seem to matter.'

'Our "Introduction to Italian" tutor refuses to assess us. He says if we did badly we'd lose interest. But all of us want to know how we're doing.'

'Everybody in our group passes everything. We're getting a bit worried.'

'We have to write our own assessment of ourselves on our report forms. I never say I'm good at anything because it sounds like I'm showing off.'

'I understand all the work but I'm no good at getting it down on paper.'

'Our teacher sets our exam paper. But, of all the topics she revised, only one came up.'

'We do a lot of presentations, which I reckon is unfair as some people are more extrovert than others.'

'We took the exam at the end of the course, so, by the time the teacher discovered I hadn't understood a lot, it was too late.'

'My work experience supervisor resented having me foisted on him, so when my college tutor visited me and asked him how I was doing he dropped me in it.'

'I got confused by all the possible answers in the multiple choice test so I just started guessing.'

Under the pressure of day-to-day teaching and training it's easy to forget the power and significance of assessment for ourselves when setting assessment tasks for our students. We can also be tempted to include assessment automatically in our programme of work without considering its appropriateness or the way in which it will affect individual or group learning.

Task 6.3: Why assess?

Choose one of the assessment examples from Task 6.2.

- Why did you assess at this particular moment? To check learning, because of awarding body requirements, the structure of the course (end of a module or unit), institutional demands?
- Why did you choose this form of assessment? Is it easy to use, prescribed by the awarding body?
- What feedback was there to students? How was it done? How will it help them to learn?
- What action will be taken as a result of assessment? Will you cover the same content in a different way? Will individual students get particular attention?

One reason for our positive and negative experiences could be that the assessment itself didn't measure what it was intended to, or was invalid. So, a written exam is an invalid test of the ability to speak a language. A conversation with a native speaker would be more valid. More valid still, arguably, would be the ability to perform a range of oral tasks in a variety of contexts. Experienced drivers often claim the driving test to be an invalid means of assessing the ability to drive, suggesting the test is only a valid means of assessing the ability to pass the test itself! The introduction of a written test to supplement the practical driving test was criticized by some as an invalid method of assessing knowledge and awareness that is only demonstrable in real driving conditions.

Those unfortunate enough to take a driving test on several occasions should, all things being equal, have the same chance of passing it each time, since the examiners base their judgements on a series of objectively demonstrated practical skills. The test, then, is reliable. It could be made more reliable if the same skills were required to be demonstrated on more than one occasion to several examiners, thus, for example, making examinees' nerves and any individual examiner's subjectivity less influential.

Task 6.4: Rating assessment methods

Table 6.1 shows a series of learning tasks and the method selected to assess each one. Decide, with a colleague, using a scale of 0–5, where 0 is low and 5 is high, how you would rate the methods in each case for both validity and reliability.

Table 6.1 Rating methods of assessment

Learning	Assessment method	Validity	Reliability
The causes of the First World War	Essay		
Empathizing with the emotional problems of 16-year-olds	Multiple choice test		
Memorizing chemical elements	Short answer questions		
Metaphor patterns in *Antony and Cleopatra*	Open book exam (text taken into exam and used for reference)		
Dribbling in football	Skills test		
Typical high-street shopping habits	Assignment/research task		
Knowledge of road signs	Written test		
Improving accent in a foreign language	Peer assessment		
Using 'Table' in Microsoft Word	Self-assessment		
Punctuation	Oral exam		
General receptionist duties	Discussion		
Dealing with customer complaints	Role-play		
Domestic mobility for the physically disabled	Case study of physically disabled client		

Satterly (1990: 224, original emphasis) points out that validity and invalidity aren't absolute qualities of assessment: '... one cannot meaningfully talk of an assessment or test being valid or invalid, but only of its *interpretation* as valid or invalid *for some specified purpose'*.

Task 6.5

Where validity or reliability was low in the examples above, how could you increase it, or what other method would be a more valid or reliable one?

A valid assessment method is one which tests whether the aims and objectives of a learning experience have been achieved. Discussion with a student would have a fairly low validity rating where general receptionist duties were concerned. Much more valid would be observation by a tutor in a real or simulated situation with a structured checklist or questionnaire relating to the skills and abilities specified in aims and objectives such as handling phone calls and dealing with clients. Although an essay would have high validity in testing a student's grasp of the causes of the First World War, allowing discursive analysis of complicated processes, it could be relatively unreliable. A detailed marking scheme would increase reliability by ensuring that the same abilities and qualities were being credited for all students by all assessors.

6.3   *Referencing*

KEY ISSUES

The type of referencing we select will depend on the nature of our aims and objectives

Criterion referencing is arguably the most effective at giving a picture of learning achievement

---

To find out how effectively learning has taken place, we need to compare a performance, a demonstration of skill, knowledge or ability with something else as a way of characterizing it. This choice of a relation or correspondence is a choice of referencing type. Our selection of referencing type should follow from the aims and objectives we have set for student learning.

Should we wish to compare an individual student's achievement with that of the group she or he is a member of – whether that be a class, year group or national cohort – we would select norm referencing. The assumption here is that the performances of any group follow a normal curve of distribution – put simply, small percentages achieving high and low scores, with the majority achieving average marks. Raw scores are therefore adjusted to fit this normal curve and a picture given of any individual's performance in comparison with the group as a whole. This approach has drawn criticism from those claiming standards have fallen in public examinations. Norm referencing, they argue, bears no relation to absolute standards of achievement: should standards actually fall, grade distribution would mask this by remaining the same. Its defenders claim that it is fairer to assume a conformity of ability in successive year cohorts than exact conformity of question or overall exam paper level of difficulty. Those hostile to eleven-plus testing have argued that norm referencing allows authorities to select at random according to the resources they choose to allocate to selective education. A further argument against norm referencing challenges any claim it may make to tell us anything of value about an individual's learning achievement.

An approach that does do this, it is argued, is criterion referencing. Here the correspondence is between the performance and an objective standard or criterion. The difference between this and norm referencing can be seen in the following example: X may be regarded by all in her group as having by far the best singing voice, but measured against criteria relating to, say, enunciation, pitch, tone, interpretation and expressiveness, she may fare differently.

Task 6.6

6.6(a) Reflect on your own experience of both norm and criterion referenced assessment.

6.6(b) Compare your experiences with the rest of the group. How did they help or hinder your learning and overall educational achievement?

Criterion referencing may be combined with grade referencing, where criteria and levels of achievement relating to them are connected with points on a scale, literal or numerical. But they need not be and, as we shall see in Section 6.6, much recording of achievement in PCE is descriptive of that achievement with little or no use of grades or marks.

Other types of referencing widely used in the sector include comparisons with a scale of dependence moving to independence, and ipsative referencing, where the comparison is with own previous performances. Both of these are prominent features of assessment in special needs education.

Task 6.7

6.7(a) Choose two assessment tasks you have recently set. What type of referencing did you use in each case? Why did you choose them?

6.7(b) Share this with the rest of the group. Were particular referencing types prominent in certain subject areas or on specific courses?

The selection of referencing type is, as we mentioned earlier, connected with your aims and objectives. If, for example, a central aim was about skill development, then ipsative referencing should be part of your overall assessment. And, as we shall now see, it is your aims and objectives which should also determine the assessment techniques and strategies you use.

6.4   *Assessment techniques*

KEY ISSUES

Assessment techniques are used in specific contexts

These contexts may limit our freedom to use particular strategies

Where possible, assessment strategies should be related to the aims
and objectives of learning

Before looking at particular assessment techniques or strategies, it is worth
considering the contexts in which we intend to deploy them. Rowntree
(1987) identifies a range of assessment features or modes. Assessment is
variously formal or informal: at one extreme a degree finals paper, at the
other, very generalized judgements made by a teacher as he or she observes
an individual or group. It is formative or summative, its prime purpose
being either to support student learning or, on the other hand, to gather
information about it. It is continuous or terminal, taking place throughout a course of study or on its completion. It may focus on coursework
or examinations, concern itself with process (the learning activities of
students) or with product, something generated by that process, such as
a drawing, an essay or a display, for example. The assessment may be
internal, carried out by those within an institution or external (an examining body). Rowntree applies Hudson's (1966) distinction between con-
vergent thinking, where students excel at a rational task with a single
answer and divergent thinking, which thrives on open-ended tasks allowing creative freedom and imagination, to assessment. And finally, he describes assessment as tending to be idiographic or nomothetic – that is, either
concerned with characterizing or describing an individual's uniqueness,
or more interested in comparing individuals with others in an attempt to
arrive at a more general understanding of achievement.

Task 6.8

Consider the assessment you undertake as part of your teaching. Which
of Rowntree's features can be accurately applied to it?

We will have more or less choice as to how we assess according to the
context we work in. Our institution may, for example, prefer a particular examination board, require us to assess internally, continuously and
report achievement terminally. But, where we do have choice, both the

features of assessment and the particular strategies we use should be determined by the nature and purpose of learning, as expressed in our aims and objectives.

Task 6.9

Table 6.2 presents a set of aims with related objectives as well as a series of assessment strategies. Match the aims and objectives to the most suitable strategies.

A suggested matching for Table 6.2 is as follows:

A	8	**G**	3	**M**	11
B	17	**H**	12	**N**	10
C	15	**I**	6	**O**	14
D	13	**J**	4	**P**	7
E	1	**K**	5	**Q**	9
F	16	**L**	2		

Task 6.10

Now undertake a similar exercise with your own work. Consider the aims and objectives either of a scheme of work, a series of sessions or of a single lesson. Look at the strategies you use to assess learning. How far do your strategies match your aims and objectives? Are there more suitable techniques you might use?

We have seen above that there can be at least two reasons for our use of some assessment strategies rather than others: a syllabus or our institution may require us to follow a particular pattern of assessment; or certain strategies may be more or less appropriate for the learning we wish our students to experience – that is, they fit our aims and objectives. But there are other reasons why teachers use particular assessment techniques and not others.

Task 6.11

Choose three assessment strategies you use frequently and and three you never use. Apart from the two reasons specified above, are there further reasons for your using or not using those you have chosen?

Table 6.2 Choosing suitable assessment strategies

Aims	Objectives	Strategies
A To exercise overall command of emergency services throughout a major incident	Maintain clear and accurate communications through changing circumstances	1 Objective/multiple choice test
B To reflect on clinical practice	Evaluate positive and negative aspects of interactions with patients	2 Self-assessment
C To handle TV interviews effectively	Demonstrate an ability to use appropriate body language on camera	3 Demonstration of skills/routine (e.g. resuscitation)
D To be aware of a range of sources of information	Search the library catalogue by author, subject or title	4 Examination consisting of long essays
E To develop and retain knowledge of costs of building materials	Know the costs of a variety of types of bricks	5 Role-play
F To understand the meaning of vocabulary	Define key words in a given passage	6 Interview
G To bring about an awareness of health and safety matters	Indicate where fire exits are	7 Group discussion
H To deal with major technical malfunctions	Describe action which would cancel or override malfunctions	8 Simulation exercise
I To converse fluently in Spanish	Conduct a one-to-one conversation about everyday topics	9 Display
J To identify major literary themes	Trace and describe ideas of kingship in Shakespeare's history plays	10 Short answer test
K To be able to support clients in expressing their emotions	Draw out clients' feelings about a traumatic incident	11 Seminar presentation
L To monitor own progress	Aware of level of own achievement	12 Problem-solving exercise
M To develop an argument and defend own views	Present an analysis of the causes of inflation and respond to questions from colleagues	13 Information gathering exercise
N To understand the structure of the British constitution	Describe broadly the functions of executive, legislature and judiciary	14 Peer assessment
O To be able to give positive feedback	Appraise colleagues' work without giving rise to animosity	15 Audio/videotaping
P To develop the capacity to work as a member of team	Contribute ideas to a team project	16 Comprehension test
Q To develop a sense of design	Able to use colour, shape and image to present a concept visually	17 Log/diary

When we conducted Task 6.11 with Certificate of Education students, the following reasons came up most frequently. Time constraints often preclude the use of more elaborate assessment – teachers are often wary of allowing the assessment tail to wag the learning dog. Teachers themselves admit to lacking confidence in their skills to devise and use particular strategies, particularly more complex ones such as role-play. Others doubt whether students themselves have the skills to deal with the demands of specific strategies, such as peer assessment. Many teachers feel they lack the resources to use certain techniques, for example, access to a video camera, a library or a PC. Teachers can be deterred by the comparative difficulty of some strategies – a log or diary are often cited – where they feel complex, often subjective judgements are required of them and there is the associated problem of reporting such achievement to third parties.

One of the reasons above mentions student skills. We saw in Chapter 3 how particular learning strategies suit some individuals rather more than others; similarly, individuals find that particular assessment strategies allow them to perform to their maximum potential and differentiation in assessment, even when the same learning, the same knowledge or skills acquisition is being tested, offers them the flexibility to be able to do just this. Differentiation may mean selecting different assessment methods for different groups, or alternative tasks and questions within a given assessment exercise. Certificate of Education students have given the following examples of how they have used differentiation in their assessment:

- men and women were placed in single-sex groups for a simulation exercise on a management course, when it was discovered that men in mixed-sex groups dominated the organization of the task, relegating the women to secondary roles;
- on a floristry course, some students with limited literary ability were examined for part of their assessment by oral interview;
- in a comprehension exercise, assessment material was provided using examples relating to students' ethnic or cultural background;
- numeracy test papers were set in a student's first language.

Task 6.12

6.12(a) Differentiation often raises the issue of equal opportunities. Discuss the examples above in your group. Do they give the students concerned a more equal opportunity of having their knowledge and skills properly assessed or an unfair advantage over others?

6.12(b) Do you use differentiation in your assessment? Do you now feel there are situations where you could and should use it?

6.5 *Competence-based assessment*

The development of competence-based assessment has grown from changes in both work-related and vocational education and training. A range of education initiatives in the 1980s, such as the Certificate of Pre-vocational Education (CPVE) and the Technical and Vocational Education Initiative (TVEI), attempted to broaden the academic, subject-centred secondary and FE curricula to provide opportunities for learning and achievement for the many such curricula excluded. Out of these initiatives grew the GNVQ, but agreement on the nature and relationship of the general and vocational elements of post-14 education is far from being reached (for a detailed treatment of 'Vocationalism', see Chapter 1). However, such a broadening of the curriculum required assessment that was more flexible and equipped to measure a much wider range of demonstrated ability than previously. At the same time, new approaches to the assessment of work-based training were pioneered in the succession of initiatives launched to combat the spiralling youth unemployment of the early 1980s. As these developed, they became the template for a much broader range of work-based assessment strategies as the structural changes in the economy, such as the expansion of the service sector and the contraction of manufacturing, meant that a workforce was required which was more flexible and adaptable, equipped with generic, transferable skills rather than specific skills limited to a narrow occupational role. There was also disenchantment with the capacity of existing vocational qualifications to guarantee the ability to perform occupational tasks satisfactorily at work and to offer the opportunities for development and progression. The review of the National Council for Vocational Qualifications (NCVQ) led to a framework of NVQs with occupational standards set by 'industry lead bodies'.

There are four major issues at the centre of the debate about competence-based assessment. The first concerns charges that it is unable to distinguish between levels of performance. Competencies cannot be graded: you are either competent at something or you are not. You can't be 'very', 'fairly', or 'just about' competent! Critics argue that motivation is therefore affected; there is simply no incentive for students to strive to do better, when a less thorough performance could be sufficient evidence to gain a competence. Defenders of this approach to assessment point out that it is its avoidance of grading which is its strength; that individual achievement is related to performance criteria and underpinning knowledge rather than being compared to the achievement of other students or some absolute, unattainable standard.

The second issue concerns the extent to which competencies focus on the performance or behavioural aspects of learning, rather than, say, cognitive aspects which are not so easily demonstrable publicly. While some may be happy with this focus for more obviously skill-based learning, it is argued that its application is inappropriate to professional contexts which require greater knowledge and understanding, such as nurse

Figure 6.2 Examples of competencies used to assess a Post-compulsory Certificate of Education course

---

Core competence: demonstrate within a teaching programme practical presentation skills, flexible modes of delivery, awareness of social and cultural issues and skill in classroom management.
Specific competencies:
1 can use a variety of teaching approaches, methods and strategies appropriate to learners' needs;
2 can manage a variety of learning environments to the optimum advantage of learners;
3 can demonstrate a range of communication skills and techniques which meet learners' needs (including non-verbal);
4 can demonstrate and create positive attitudes towards equal opportunities in a variety of learning situations;
5 can demonstrate an awareness of stereotyping, labelling and rule-making and their significance in learning situations.

---

education, social-work training, teacher education or police training. Many Post-compulsory Certificate in Education courses are now assessed using a competence-based approach. The competencies shown in Figure 6.2 are examples from one such course.

Task 6.13: Sufficient evidence?

In pairs, specify the evidence you think would be sufficient for the demonstration of each of the five competencies shown in Figure 6.2. As a group, to what extent was the public demonstration alone considered sufficient evidence?

Even though these five competencies are concerned with classroom practice and therefore appear to be performance orientated, it is likely that each needed supplementary evidence. We can observe (1) teaching approaches, methods and strategies but how do we judge if they are appropriate to learners' needs? Equally, we can observe a teacher establish and operate a rule (5), but how are we to know if they are themselves aware of the rule's significance in learning situations? The relationship between knowledge and performance has been considered in some detail (see Wolf and Black 1990) with some arguing that knowledge evidence waters down competence-based assessment, since assessing performance should equally be an assessment of any knowledge underpinning it. On the other hand, three major enquiries into post-16 qualifications have highlighted the importance of supplementing performance evidence with that from a range of other assessment strategies, particularly externally-set and marked tests (Beaumont 1995; Capey 1995; Dearing 1996).

The third issue concerns the reliability of competence-based assessment. Although, on the surface, performance criteria can be spelled out in detail, assessors' interpretation of such criteria can vary. Systems of internal and external verification do, of course, help to minimize such variation but, as Wolf (1993: 17) points out:

> the [assessment] process is complex, incremental, and, above all, *judgemental*. The performance observed – directly, or in the form of artefacts – is *intrinsically* variable: one person's playing of a piano piece, one person's essay, is by definition not exactly the same as another's, and cannot be fitted mechanistically to either a written list of criteria or an exemplar.

Task 6.14: Acceptable evidence

If possible, this exercise should be carried out in curriculum groups, or in groups of closely allied subjects (e.g. hairdressing and health and beauty). Select a task which a student would be asked to perform as a part of their assessment. If you have a common framework such as an NVQ, agree a level at which such a task would be assessed. Now, individually, try to describe – *in your own language* – not that of a set of performance criteria, and in as much detail as possible, what you would accept as performance evidence for the successful completion of this task. Compare your accounts.

Finally, some argue that a competence-based system makes learning assessment-led. That is, for students at least, one eye is always on the competencies that have yet to be awarded and the entire course of study then becomes skewed towards ticking off such competencies. This can lead to extreme behaviour illustrated by the following (true) incident which occurred on a Certificate of Education course. A college student had been knocked down by a vehicle on campus and (fortunately only slightly) injured. A Certificate of Education student, a member of college staff, had, being a first-aider, attended and dealt with the incident. Arriving late for the Certificate of Education session, he explained the reason for his lateness. The tutor made a concerned enquiry about the injured student. 'He'll be OK', was the reply, 'but what a stroke of luck! I've been waiting for something like this to come along for months to give me the evidence for that health and safety competence!'

Competence-based assessment in action

Example 6.1 presents material relating to NVQ assessment, and Example 6.2 presents material relating to GNVQ assessment. Both qualifications are divided into units which are then sub-divided into elements of competence. The NVQ unit concerns Unit E2 'Maintain the Safety of Children',

Example 6.1

Element Assessment Record Sheet

Unit N° & Title:

    E.2   **MAINTAIN THE SAFETY OF CHILDREN**

Element N° & Title:

    E.2.2   **Maintain supervision of children**

Performance Criteria N°	Log Entry N° Page N°	Log Entry N° N°	Evidence Gathering Methods
1	1	1	EA
2	1	2	A
3	4	19	A
4	3 (4)	14 (17)	A (A)
5	4	19	A
6	9	36	B

Key:
A =	Direct Observation	B =	Questioning
C =	Interrogated/ rationale	D =	Work Plans
E =	Inspection of setting	F =	Reflective accounts
G =	Log books/ diaries	H =	Plans
I =	Case studies/ assignments	J =	Child Observations
K =	Sim/ role play sk. rehearsal	L =	Analogue evidence
M =	Prior achievement		

Methods used for this element were ? (tick methods used)

Overall | A̶ | B̶ | C | D | E̶ | F | G | H | I | J | K | L | M̶ |

Knowledge | A̶ | B̶ | C | D | E̶ | F | G | H | I | J | K | L | M̶ |

Range	Log Entry N°	Evidence Gathering Methods
Location :		
indoors	38	G
outdoors.	38	G

Special Notes

    Direct observation of performance in the workplace especially with regard to E.2.2.1, E.2.2.2, E.2.2.3, E.2.2.4.

Candidate's Name : _C. Rowland_   Assessor's Name : LYNDA EVANS
                C. ROWLAND   (Please Print)

Signature : _____   Signature : Lynda Evans

© CEYA/JABS 11/03/92   Date Element Completed : 20/10/95

Example 6.1 (Cont'd)

E.2.2 Maintain supervision of children

Performance Criteria

2.2.1 The level of adult supervision agreed for the setting is maintained at all times to ensure the safety of children.

2.2.2 Supervision of children is carried out in a calm, relaxed manner and promotes children's self confidence.

2.2.3 Supervision is sufficient to identify potentially dangerous situations and appropriate action is taken to rectify them while protecting children without undermining their confidence and control.

2.2.4 Safety rules are explained to children as appropriate to their level of understanding to increase their awareness of the need for safety and supervision.

2.2.5 The extent of supervision avoids overprotection of children.

2.2.6 Policies and procedures for collecting children agreed for the setting ensure that children are not handed over without authorisation.

RANGE   Location: indoors; outdoors.

Examples and definitions to clarify terms used in the range or performance criteria.

2.2.1 Level of adult supervision includes adult/child ratio agreed for the setting.

2.2.4 Examples of safety rules: restricting access to certain areas; prohibiting actions which are liable to cause harm to other children.

2.2.5 Examples of overprotection: not allowing girls to climb; overprotection of disabled children.

EVIDENCE REQUIREMENTS – E.2.2

Performance Evidence

The preferred methods of assessment are:-

1. Direct observation of performance in the workplace especially with regard to E.2.2.1, E.2.2.2, E.2.2.3, E.2.2.4.

2. Oral questioning contingent on aspects of performance to cover performance criteria or parts of the range that are not readily observable.

3. Interrogation of candidate's rationale for activities/performance.

4. Log books or diaries of day to day practice kept for assessment purposes where appropriate including notes of safety rules, notes concerning collection of children.

5. Plans and other evidence of preparation for activities or routines.

6. Evidence of prior achievement.

Where performance is not directly observed, any evidence should be authenticated, preferably by colleagues, supervisors, parents or other appropriate person or by detailed questioning of the candidate by the assessor to establish authenticity.

Where appropriate, written and oral evidence may be supplemented by diagrams, photographs or other practical or audio visual materials.

Knowledge Evidence

Evidence of an appropriate level of knowledge and understanding in the following areas is required to be demonstrated from the above assessment process supplemented as necessary from oral or written questions or other knowledge tests or from evidence of prior learning.

E.2.2.a The regulations concerning adult/child ratios appropriate in the setting and the importance of adhering to these.

E.2.2.b That adult anxiety/inappropriate reactions to events, are often transmitted to children, and that stereotyping can prevent a child from achieving his/her potential.

E.2.2.c The importance of policies and procedures for collection of children taking account of any special circumstances e.g. Care Orders.

Example 6.1 (Cont'd)

Evidence Log Sheet

Page No 1

Entry Number &Date	Evidence Gathering Method	Entry	Unit and Element Reference
1 8/2 LE	E A	Empty hall set up as per Chris's instructions. Plenty of room between activities, tables and equipment. 20 children - 3 adults. Doors clear. Room was not too hot or cold. Natural light dull (rainy) so lights put on (her decision as leader)	E 1.1.2 E 2.2.1 E 1.1.3 E 1.1.4
2 8/2 LE	A	Chris at activity table 'tasting'. Each child given individual spoon. Discuss with children taste, colours, textures, smells. Guessing what it is. Child joins and is told to wash hands and says what about their own spoon. "If Lotty had a tummy ache she'd pass it on to…" Chris asks who would like to try.	E 2.1.1 E 2.4.4 E 2.2.2
3/4 8/2 LE	A	Child starts crying. Chris goes to where he's sitting and puts her arm round and talks reassuringly. He says he wants to do a painting. Child chooses apron. Returns to activity. Child guesses taste. Chris - "You're right G-"enthusiastically. Children in water tray - goes over and says not to splash over sides as will wet shoes and socks. Says to child to roll up sleeves - he "can't as tight" so she does. Went over and rang small bell and told children they had 5 minutes to finish what they're doing and pack toys away. Some children tidied up with adults - others finished painting activity.	E 2.4.5 E 2.2.2.
14 9/2 LE	A	Chris explains child tripped because he was running across the floor ignoring toys.	E 2.2.4 E2.2.1 RANGE (indirectly)
17 9/2 LE	A	Chris asks 2 children to play with planes on the mat (they were running round) so they wouldn't collide with furniture.	E 2.2.4 E 2.1.6
9 9/2 LE	A	Chris asks 2 boys moving garage (clearing up time) to move things out of their way	E 2.2.5 E 2.1.5 E 2.1.6

Candidate's Name: CHRIS Rowland.

and the element is 'Maintain Supervision of Children'. The Element Assessment Record Sheet (p. 143) relates the assessor's log entries of direct observation and inspection of setting to performance criteria. The six performance criteria are then set out (p. 144) as are both the methods of assessment of performance evidence and knowledge evidence. There is then a page of log entries made by the assessor (p. 145). Familiarize yourself with the material and then complete Task 6.15.

Task 6.15

Look through the assessor's log entries presenting evidence of direct observation and inspection of setting for Element 2.2. You will note that they provide evidence for performance criteria 2.2.1, 2.2.2, 2.2.3 and 2.2.4. What evidence would you look for relating to performance criteria 2.2.5 and 2.2.6 and what methods would you use to gather it?

The GNVQ material shown in Example 6.2 below is from a very different curriculum area, leisure and tourism. This is an Advanced GNVQ and the element concerned is '1.1: investigate the structure and scale of the UK leisure and tourism industries'. Page 147 shows seven performance criteria, range statements relating to them, evidence indicators, amplification and guidance. On page 148 is the assignment 'The Ownership Triangle', which will offer evidence relating to all seven performance criteria of Element 1.1. From page 149 onwards is reproduced Emma Richard's booklet relating to performance criteria 1 and 2. Finally, on page 154 is the teacher's feedback sheet.

Task 6.16

What are the main similarities and differences between NVQ and GNVQ?

Task 6.17

From the limited information available to you, how far does each piece of assessment answer criticisms of competence-based assessment that it:

• fails to distinguish levels of performance;
• focuses on performance/behaviour;
• can be unreliable;
• can be assessment-led?

Example 6.2

Element 1.1: Investigate the structure and scale of the UK leisure and tourism industries

PERFORMANCE CRITERIA

A student must:

1 describe the **structure of the UK leisure and recreation industry** and give examples of its facilities

2 describe the **structure of the UK travel and tourism industry and give examples of its facilities**

3 **assess** the **scale of the leisure and tourism industries** nationally

4 explain the **role of the public sector** and give examples of public sector organisations from both industries

5 explain the **role of the private sector** and give examples of private sector organisations from both industries

6 explain the **role of the voluntary sector** and give examples of voluntary sector organisations from both industries

7 **investigate the relationship** between the sectors

RANGE

Structure of the UK leisure and recreation industry: arts and entertainment, sports and physical activities, outdoor activities, play, heritage, catering and accommodation

Structure of the UK travel and tourism industry:

travel services (retail travel agencies, business travel agencies, tour operators, principals),

tourism (national tourist boards, regional tourist boards, tourist information centres, tourist attractions, guiding services, currency exchange, accommodation, catering, transport)

Assess in relation to: economy, employment

Scale of the leisure and tourism industries: numbers employed nationally, contribution to the national economy, contribution to the balance of payments

Role of the public sector: national provision, local provision; policy setting, policy implementing, contract management, funding, providing facilities; joint provision

Role of the private sector: providing facilities, managing facilities; financial return on investment; risk ventures; joint provision

Role of the voluntary sector: influencing national policy, organising national interest; developing facilities, managing facilities; organising local interest, providing for a common interest; raising funds

Investigate the relationship in terms of: dual use, joint provision, partnership, contracting, co-operative ventures

EVIDENCE INDICATORS

A report outlining in general terms the structure and scale of the UK leisure and tourism industries. The report should give a broad description of the structure of both industries supported by examples of their facilities. Sufficient examples should be given to cover the entire breadth of each industry as listed in the range 'Structure' for that industry.

The report should also assess the scale of the two industries nationally and explain the roles of each of the three sectors using examples from both industries. Sufficient examples should be given to reflect all aspects of their roles as listed in the range 'Role' for each sector. The report should also include the findings of an investigation into the relationship between the three sectors.

AMPLIFICATION

Structure of the UK leisure and recreation industry (PC1) the categories given in the range are broad categories reflecting the breadth of the industry. The categories provide students with a framework for analysing the industry. The facilities that students observe often cover more than one category, e.g. a leisure centre can provide indoor sports facilities, outdoor activities and catering facilities.

Scale of the leisure and tourism industries (PC3) figures are likely to be imprecise, particularly in relation to parts of the leisure and recreation industry, but the most recent figures (usually about two years in arrears) should be used to give students a broad picture of the scale and importance of these industries.

Role of the public sector and role of the private sector (PC4 and PC5) as a result of compulsory competitive tendering (CCT) the roles of the public and private sectors are becoming more interdependent.

Investigate the relationship (PC7) the concepts listed in the range, like joint provision and dual use, can be applied to all sectors from both industries.

GUIDANCE

Students may develop understanding of the two industries by sharing their experiences of leisure and recreation and of travel and tourism in group discussions. This understanding may be further developed by using appropriate information sources both inside and outside school or college.

Teachers and tutors should ensure that the full breadth of both industries is covered.

Teachers and tutors should be aware of publications available from organisations such as National Tourist Boards, Regional Tourist Boards, Sports Council and General Household Survey.

Example 6.2 (Cont'd)

> GNVQ ADVANCED
> LEISURE AND TOURISM

THE OWNERSHIP TRIANGLE

AIMS

The aim of this assignment is to enable the student to investigate the structure and scale of the leisure and tourism industry.

OBJECTIVES

The successful completion of this assignment will enable the student to claim from Mandatory Unit 1: Investigating the leisure and tourism industries, Element 1:1 pc 1, 2, 3, 4, 5, 6 and 7. All students are reminded to read carefully the specification and to make sure that all relevant aspects of the range are covered.

PART ONE

Following the lessons on the structure of the leisure and tourism industry, compile a **booklet** which outlines the structure of each of the components within the two industries. Your booklet should be word-processed and illustrated in your IT lessons and should include examples of facilities to highlight your comments.

PART TWO

Write a short **report** on the scale of the leisure and tourism industries in terms of the economy and the number of people employed. You should try to put forward an argument in support of the industries as important to our economy and include any relevant figures to support your argument.

PART THREE

In order to show your understanding of the ownership and managing of leisure and tourism facilities you should hand-write an **essay** which should be titled 'Public, Private, Voluntary – can they work together?' In your essay you should define the role of each sector, giving examples of facilities in each sector and completing the worksheets from class visits and then explain how the three sectors work together.

Example 6.2 (Cont'd)

The Ownership Triangle

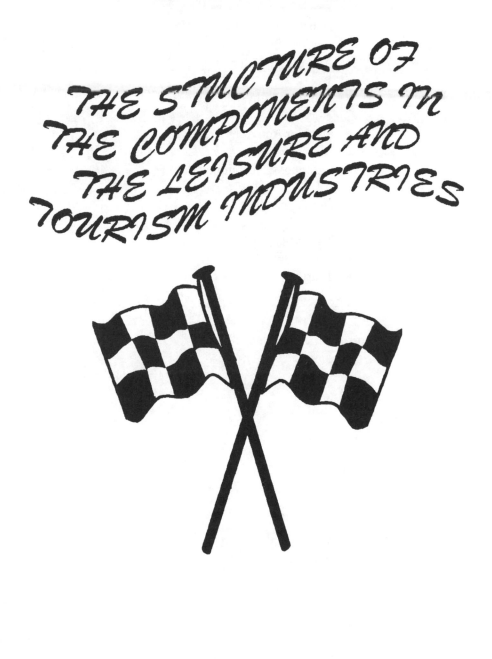

Example 6.2 (Cont'd)

<u>Contents</u>

- Department of National Heritage

- Arts & Entertainment

- Sports and Physical Activities

- Outdoor Activities

- Catering & Accommodation

- Heritage

- Travel Services

- Tourism

Example 6.2 (Cont'd)

Department of National Heritage

The Department of National Heritage was formed by the Government in order to oversee the running of the leisure and tourism industry. At the head of the department is a full Cabinet Minister, the Secretary of State for National Heritage who at the present time is Virginia Bottomley. The department is responsible to the government for all activity within the industry. It controls the many stationary bodies set up to regulate the industry such as the BTA, the Arts Council and the Sports Council.
Departments within the Department of National Heritage are:

- Libraries, Galleries and Museums Group

- Arts, Sport and Lottery Group

- Broadcasting and Media Group

- Royal Parks Agency

- Heritage and Tourism Group

- Historic Royal Palaces Agency

Government money comes to leisure and tourism through the Department of National Heritage, and they are influenced by the government when making policies.

Example 6.2 (Cont'd)

Arts & Entertainment

In the public sector is the Arts Council of Great Britain. It took over the work of the Council for the Encouragement of Music and the Arts which was formed in 1946. The Council was re-formed under its present name in 1964 and operates under Royal Charter. It's main objectives are to:

a) develop and improve the knowledge, understanding and practice of the arts.

b) increase the accessibility of the arts to the public throughout Great Britain.

c) advise and co-operate with the departments of Government, local authorities and others.

They receive funding from Central Government and the National Lottery. Each local authority will have an 'arts department', and there will be arts development officers who may fund visiting performers. They work with the local community on special projects.

In the voluntary sector at a national level the National Trust is the only main national organisation along with the Scout and Guide movement for arts and entertainment. It crosses over with heritage. At a local level there are small groups of local people who participate in specific arts and entertainment. For example, amateur dramatic groups, choral groups and dance classes.

In the private sector at a national level the majority of arts and entertainment facilities are provided by private companies. They earn large amounts of revenue, and are companies such as the Rank Organisation, First Leisure, Granada, Whitbread, Virgin and Warners. At a local level there are a few privately owned theatres, galleries and cinemas.

Example 6.2 (Cont'd)

Catering & Accommodation

The catering facilities in the UK today cover the preparation, distribution and serving of food and drink. Some examples of private sector facilities (companies providing products and services in order to generate a financial profit) are: restaurants, cafes, fast food outlets, public houses and motorway services. Some examples of public sector facilities (owned by central or local government, often run at a loss - subsidised) are: contract catering services such as Chartwell's cafe in Orpington college, and the Walnuts Leisure Centre cafe. Some examples of voluntary sector facilities (generally non-profit-making dependent on volunteers often serving special needs and interest groups, breaking even) are: Meals on wheels provided by the WRVS, Salvation Army and catering facilities within sports clubs.

Accommodation in the UK today can be classified as commercial or non-commercial, serviced or self catering, urban or rural and static or mobile. Some examples of private sector accommodation include: hotels (which can be part of a franchise and parts of larger groups or small and individual), motels, lodges, cottages/chalets, farm guest houses, B&B's, caravan/camp sites, holiday camps, time share and VFR (visiting friends and relatives). Some examples of public sector accommodation are: caravan/camp sites. Some examples of voluntary sector accommodation are; youth hostels and the YMCA/YWCA.

All of the facilities are graded by regulatory organisations such as the ETB. They are not only graded on the quality of the place, but also on the range of facilities/services you can expect. The more crowns etc. given, the higher the quality and the wider the range of facilities offered. Hotels, guest houses, inns, B&B's and farm houses are all graded by crowns. Lodges (motorway stopovers) are graded by moons. Self catering holiday homes are graded by keys. Caravan, chalet or camping parks are graded by Q's, and all of the accommodation is graded on how accessible it is to wheelchair users. Other forms of grading are also used such as stars, and some Tour Operators have their own regulating system.

Example 6.2 (Cont'd)

FEEDBACK SHEET
(GRADING)

Advanced GNVQ - Leisure and Tourism

GRADING THEMES	MERIT	DISTINCTION
1 PLANNING - DRAWING UP PLANS		
2 PLANNING - MONITORING ACTION		
3 INFORMATION SEEKING - USING SOURCE	✓	
4 INFORMATION SEEKING - ESTABLISH VALIDITY	✓	
5 EVALUATION - EVALUATING OUTCOMES		
6 EVALUATION - JUSTIFYING APPROACH		
7 QUALITY OF OUTCOMES - SYNTHESIS		✓
8 QUALITY OF OUTCOMES - COMMAND OF LANGUAGE		✓

Tutor Comments:

An excellent piece of work - well done, Emma.   Can you just add the heritage worksheet?

You have the potential to achieve the highest grades but you must provide more evidence of how you planned and monitored the assignment.

Your evaluation is good but it needs to include alternatives you could have used and more justification for your approach.

Overall - very promising for the future if you maintain this standard

ASSESSOR SIGNATURE_ J. De Silva ___ STUDENT SIGNATURE_ E. Richards

It is likely that the professional skills required by teachers new to competence-based assessment are in two areas: first in devising and using strategies which produce the appropriate evidence to indicate competence and second in judging whether such evidence is acceptable.

Task 6.18: Devising assessment

In the same curriculum groups as Task 6.14, specify between two and five performance criteria (use Examples 6.1 and 6.2 as a guide if necessary). Now devise the strategies you would use which together could generate sufficient evidence to indicate competence with relation to all your criteria.

Some of the questions which frequently arise with regard to devising competence-based assessment and judging the acceptability of evidence are as follows:

- are witness statements acceptable alone as third-party evidence or do they always need further verification?
- should self-assessment be corroborated by supplementary evidence?
- how many times and in how many contexts should a skill be performed to establish a competence, bearing in mind that range statements and evidence indicators offered as guidance often specify content alone?
- how far is jointly authored/produced work acceptable as evidence?
- for how many competencies can any one piece of evidence be acceptable?
- to what extent is a demonstration of competence dependent on the assessor's skill rather than the candidate's ability (in, say, a carefully managed review of progress)?

Task 6.19

How important were any of the above issues when you undertook Task 6.18? Were there any further issues which arose for your group?

6.6 Reviewing, recording and reporting achievement

The development of new courses involving a wider range of teaching and learning strategies is requiring teachers to be involved in much more complex assessment procedures. The Training and Development Award, D32, for example, asks that assessors, among other things:

- negotiate an assessment plan;
- discuss this plan;
- allow the candidate to express views/participate;
- document the process of evidence collection;
- give feedback which is specific, constructive and supportive;
- use questions which are open, clear and justifiable, not leading, probing or searching.

There is recognition here that assessment is more than an isolated judgement of a specific performance; that it should be integrated into a system of reviewing, recording and reporting achievement which teacher and student are at the centre of.

Task 6.20

6.20(a) Working in pairs, choose a recent piece of assessable coursework each of you has completed. With one of you as the student and the other as the tutor, assess the work and record your interaction involving all the D32 skills listed above. Then swap roles and repeat the exercise.

6.20(b) Which stage of the process proved the most difficult?

Many teachers find giving feedback the most problematic area of reviewing learning. This could be for a number of reasons: the tutor has the difficult task of bringing together a range of evidence of performance which she or he may not have assessed themselves; balancing feedback which is constructive and supportive while at the same time an accurate reflection of achievement is far from straightforward; negotiation assumes equality between participants when, in truth, the trainer rather than the candidate is finally empowered to make a decision about the acceptability of evidence. Francis and Young (1979), and others, have specified features which tend to characterize the giving of effective feedback. Good feedback is:

- clear and direct, whereby the reasons for assessment decisions are fully explained in language which is direct and unambiguous rather than vague or beating about the bush;
- constructive, because it is important to offer advice for further action which is in the student's capacity to take;
- descriptive of what the tutor has seen/observed/thinks rather than over-evaluative or judgemental;
- helpful and supportive on the tutor's part (this attitude must be fully communicated to the student);
- well-timed, being given as soon as is practicable after evidence has been demonstrated and at a time when the student is receptive to feedback;

- fully understood by the student, with the tutor making every effort to ensure this, leaving no unresolved questions, misunderstandings or confusions;
- specific, being related to particular incidents or learning events.

Task 6.21

How far could the features above be applied to your pair work in Task 6.20?

The recording and reporting of achievement is usually based on records or profiles which vary in structure and style. Often, an awarding body will prescribe its own format but there may be institutional, departmental or curriculum area profile reports which are related to this or are free-standing. Most are variations of the four profile formats considered below.

The graded scale

These can take a variety of forms but their common feature is their placing of performances somewhere on a given scale. In Table 6.3 the assessor ticks a box on the continuum between one pole and another.

In Table 6.4 the assessor inserts a number signifying a level of achievement for each assessment, where 1 equals good, 2 equals adequate and 3 equals poor.

Table 6.3 Polar graded scale for communication skills

Writes precisely, clearly with few errors						Expression is vague, difficult to understand with frequent errors
Written accounts are comprehensive and coherent						Written accounts are brief and bitty
Etc.						Etc.

Table 6.4 Numerical graded scale for communication skills

	1st assessment	2nd assessment	3rd assessment	4th assessment	5th assessment
Precision and clarity in writing					
Comprehensiveness of written accounts					
Etc.					

Table 6.5 Grid profile for communication skills

Written communications	Can express and reply to simple information	Can express and reply to simple information in a variety of contexts	Can express and reply to complex information	✓	Can express and reply to complex information in a variety of contexts	
Oral communications						

The strengths of the graded scale are:

- it is visually straightforward and easy to read;
- it can indicate progress when used formatively;
- it refers to specific skills/abilities.

Weaknesses include:

- the difficulty of representing precisely two ends of a real continuum by the descriptors at each pole;
- the absence of any criteria which might help the learner understand the basis of grading;
- a tendency to use ipsative referencing in the absence of assessment criteria.

Grid profiles

Grid profiles share a visual simplicity with graded scales but attempt to relate performance to assessment criteria, as shown in Table 6.5.

The advantages of grid profiles are:

- they are quick to complete;
- they specify what a student can do;
- they can be used formatively to plot development.

Disadvantages are:

- the descriptors may not do justice to learner achievement (a student who is outstanding at handling enquiries in reception might nevertheless have a tick only in the first box);
- grids are not tailored to individual students.

Open portrayals

This is essentially a blank sheet of paper on which an assessor is free to write what he or she chooses to. In practice, some are more open than others. The NVQ comments on page 145, although representing an open portrayal are closely related to a particular piece of work. A summative report at the end of a college year or course may offer a much wider portrayal.

The strengths of open portrayals are:

- they are highly dedicated to individual students;
- they are informative;
- they are comprehensive;

Weaknesses include:

- tutors have a habit of wanting to fill blank space if it exists;
- they can be unstructured;
- they can be time-consuming both to write and to read.

Criterion-referenced competence statements

This is an approach now widely adopted in PCE. The strengths of an approach using such statements are:

- they are positive, framed in 'can-do' statements;
- they lend themselves to negotiation and the reviewing of learning;
- they are related to learning/performance evidence.

Weaknesses include:

- relating evidence to competencies can be complex and time-consuming;
- there is no opportunity for levels of achievement to be acknowledged;
- learning outside the scope of particular competencies is not credited.

Many teachers working in PCE express two major anxieties about assessing their students: first, they are concerned about the increasing prominence of assessment and the time devoted to it often at the expense, they feel, of student learning; second, they worry that much assessment they are required to carry out does not do justice to the richness of the learning experience they know their students have undergone. We hope this chapter has helped them to reflect on these matters and deal with them more effectively in practice.

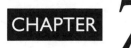

7

EXPLORING THE
CURRICULUM

7.1 What is Chapter 7 about?

For many of us, working as busy teachers and trainers in a variety of organizations, scheduled to work with the maximum number of students in the minimum amount of time, the 'curriculum' is all too often simply whatever course we happen to be teaching at the time! This chapter provides an opportunity to pause and consider just what our courses are really about. Remember, unless we really know the answer to this question, that is, understand what it is we are meant to be doing and why, how can we be sure that what we are doing is the best for our students?

In order to understand how the chapter is organized, compare a course to a building. Consider what needs to be done before starting to build a new building or prior to adding an extension to an existing building. Sections 7.2, 7.3 and 7.4 will pose some fundamental questions about the nature and organization of our courses in order to expose their foundations, rather as structural surveys and groundworks expose the fundamental state of the ground and dictate the foundations required to build a new structure or an extension.

Section 7.5 is the tea break, giving you some time to stop and consider your position in the light of all this new information before moving on to Chapter 8 which will help you to design, build and evaluate your new or revised course.

7.2 *What is the curriculum?*

KEY ISSUES

What is the curriculum and who dictates it?

Why is it continually changing?

Should it be continually changing?

As professionals working in the post-compulsory sector, we teach and train through many different courses covering a huge variety of subject matter and areas of skill development. However, one thing we have in common is that we all have some kind of curriculum through which we aim to help our students to learn.

> **Task 7.1: What is this notion of curriculum all about?**
>
> Drawing on your own experience and subject expertise, take a moment to think and then jot down a sentence explaining your own definition of 'curriculum'. Figure 7.1 shows some writers', teachers' and trainers' responses to this question.

> **Task 7.2: Comparing definitions**
>
> 7.2(a) Which, if any, of the definitions presented in Figure 7.1 fits most closely with your own ideas?
>
> 7.2(b) What are the key differences and similarities when compared to your definition?

Figure 7.1 presents a diverse set of definitions but here is one view of the key similarities and differences. See how it compares with your responses to Task 7.2. Definitions 1 and 3 emphasize teacher and trainer planning while 10 mentions planning across an organization. Definitions 2, 5 and 12 also have an institutional emphasis but 4 is the only one which explicitly mentions subjects and skills although these must be implicit in many of the others. Definition 6 and 12 provide an interesting contrast in that 12 only mentions the planned curriculum whereas 6

Figure 7.1 Some definitions of curriculum

1 The curriculum is what happens to students because of what teachers/trainers do.

2 The curriculum is a formal course of study as at a college, university or training institution.

3 The curriculum is a teacher's or trainer's intention or educational plan.

4 The curriculum is a group of subjects and/or skills which make up a programme of study.

5 The curriculum is a formal, timetabled programme of lessons.

6 The curriculum is everything that happens to students at a college, university or training organization.

7 The curriculum is an attempt to communicate the essential principles and features of an educational proposal.

8 The curriculum describes the results of instruction.

9 The curriculum lays down what's to be covered and to some extent the teaching and learning methods to be used.

10 The curriculum is the organization's plan to guide learning towards pre-specified learning outcomes.

11 The curriculum is a structured series of intended learning outcomes.

12 The curriculum consists of every learning experience planned and provided by the organization to help pupils attain learning outcomes.

13 The curriculum is the public form of attempting to put an educational idea into practice.

14 The curriculum is a menu presented to students for consumption.

includes the totality of a student's experience at an institution, the planned and the unplanned, recalling the notion of a hidden curriculum (Jackson 1968). Definitions 8, 10, 11 and 12 are similar in that all make particular mention of learning outcomes. Definition 9 alone seems to hint at ideas of curriculum content and process and 14 is unique in presenting learners as explicitly passive consumers of the curriculum. Finally, both 7 and 13 mention the notion of the curriculum as conveying a particular vision of learning while 13 emphasizes the public nature of a curriculum once it is in place.

From this, it's possible to identify what seem to be some key issues to consider in any definition of curriculum and these are shown in Figure 7.2.

This section has begun to expose and consider our own ideas about curriculum. What does some of the literature on curriculum tell us? Goodson (1994) makes the interesting point that, while curriculum development and implementation have been written about by many people, the more fundamental issues of curriculum definition, who constructs it, why and for whom have been more neglected. However, one writer who

Figure 7.2 Some key issues in defining 'curriculum'

- Evidence of planning (on a variety of scales) for student learning;
- statements of what's to be learned;
- indications of how it's to be learned;
- pointers as to the outcomes of this learning;
- statements on the role of learners in all this;
- explanations about the vision behind the curriculum;
- some dissemination or publication showing the public nature of the formal curriculum.

did address these questions was Stenhouse (1975) who starts by quoting the *Shorter Oxford English Dictionary* which defines curriculum as 'a course: especially a regular course of study as at a school or university'. Thus, curriculum may be viewed as the planned intentions of government and of teachers/trainers in their organizations. These plans often take the form of a public, written prescription and Stenhouse goes on to mention that in many countries the curriculum is a state-controlled, legal requirement. For many of us, this resembles the National Curriculum and A-level syllabuses for schools, NVQ specifications for vocational qualifications and the police and nurse training programmes all of which can be viewed as public, published documents. Indeed, Higham *et al.* (1996) portray the 16–19 curriculum for schools and colleges as simply comprising the courses or qualifications (academic, vocational and core/key skills) for which students are studying.

A second view of curriculum outlined by Stenhouse (1975) asks us to concentrate not just on the planned curriculum but on the reality of teaching and learning for teachers and students. That is, Stenhouse challenges us to view the curriculum as what really happens in our classrooms and training areas. He also points out that the key reason teachers and trainers need to study the curriculum is to examine this balance between intentions and realities and use this information to improve their work and enhance students' learning.

Taylor and Richards (1985), on the other hand, have little patience with any of the broader definitions of curriculum which try to include all the planned experiences, not just the formal things to be learned. They see these as the context within which the curriculum operates and which can affect the curriculum:

'. . . the course of study to be followed in becoming educated' is in fact the oldest known meaning of the word [curriculum]. In contemporary writings, however, the phrase is frequently translated into 'the subjects to be studied' or 'the educational experiences to be provided' and not infrequently into 'the actual subject matter to be covered'.

(Taylor and Richards 1985: 3)

Taylor and Richards argue that each of these definitions has its uses depending primarily on the context to which it is applied. Thus, a nursery curriculum might be better viewed as educational experiences such as the sand tray, a school curriculum might consist largely of subjects, whereas in post-compulsory education and training the curriculum is more closely associated with courses of study. The key issue, they say, is to choose whichever definition seems most appropriate and use this consistently and accurately.

So, bearing in mind Goodson's (1994) cautionary note, both Stenhouse (1975) and Taylor and Richards (1985) present notions of curriculum as public plans (often written) about what is to be learned and this is reflected by Higham *et al.*'s (1996) more recent contribution. However, Stenhouse adds a further idea, that of curriculum as the reality of learning for teacher and student. Whatever definition we choose to use, Taylor and Richards emphasize the need to be consistent and accurate in our use of the term 'curriculum'.

Task 7.3: Do you agree?

Set your original definition of a curriculum against those above. Where you stand now? Why do you believe this?

Having arrived at a working notion of curriculum, ask yourself a question. How much curriculum change has taken place in the last few years? The answer, of course, is that a tremendous amount has altered.

Task 7.4: Curriculum change in your work

In your own specialist area, note down the key changes you know about that have taken place in recent years. Include both the large-scale changes, often imposed by others, and the smaller-scale changes you, your colleagues or your organization have introduced.

Figure 7.3 presents a few examples of large-scale curriculum change. See if any of these figure in your list. These are curriculum developments on a national scale but interestingly, it is relatively easy to produce such a list without too much searching of the archives. The amount and rate of change in the last 15 years of the century has been remarkable. Of course, curriculum development has always taken place on a smaller scale. No doubt you will have been able to recall instances of specific course developments in your own work and organization. All this begs two key questions. Jot down your responses to Task 7.5 before reading on.

Figure 7.3 Examples of large-scale curriculum change

- schools have had several versions of the National Curriculum to contend with since 1988;
- all A levels are being reviewed in depth during the mid- to late 1990s for virtually the first time since being introduced in the early 1950s;
- GNVQs were introduced in 1992 and have been subject to ongoing development ever since;
- vocational qualifications are in the process of being transformed by the steady introduction of NVQs, first devised in 1988 and revised throughout the late 1990s;
- national police training was completely revised in the mid-1980s and further changes are planned for the late 1990s;
- nurse training was radically altered in the late 1980s and developments in both this and associated areas of medical training have continued ever since.

Task 7.5: What do you think?

7.5(a) Just why does the curriculum change?

7.5(b) Should it be continually developing?

At this point, many teachers and trainers might well be tempted to mutter something about the government (or whichever agency is in overall charge of their area of work) never seeming to provide enough time or resources to do a proper job, never allowing enough time to allow any change to settle down before introducing yet more alterations and, perhaps, never really seeming to know what they really do want! In particular instances, this might well be true. Indeed, some writers such as Ahier and Ross (1995) talk about curriculum being the result of a creative tension. Think of the haggling you can see taking place in many market-places abroad when you're on holiday. Seller and prospective buyer engage in a process of bargaining (arguing, debating, sometimes almost coming to blows!) until, if it works out, a compromise is reached. Each is out to get what they want. This is another form of creative tension and many curricula are the final outcome of argument, debate and conflict over different ideas about what should be taught and learned, how this should take place and the best means of assessing learning. Thus, all present curricula could be represented as simply the best compromise (hopefully) or the least bad compromise (more realistically) that can be achieved until new knowledge and ideas, together with evaluation data, make a revision necessary.

More cynically, the bargaining might be distorted by one of the hag-
glers threatening to use physical force whereupon the other calls her or
his friends over to help! Thus, in this view, the curricula many of us have
to deal with at present might simply be a dominant power group's position which will be replaced as soon as the balance of power shifts, with
less importance being attached to the quality of education and training
involved than to the political kudos attached to having produced change.
The work of Ball (1987) and Goodson and Hargreaves (1996) largely on
schools, and of Hyland (1994) on NVQs, all provide some fascinating
insights into the politics of curriculum change but perhaps it might all be
summarized by someone writing much earlier.

Taba (1962) was moved to use the term 'tinkering' when she portrayed
curriculum as being the result of constant and ongoing modification.
Think of 'tinkering' and imagine when you have been endlessly trying to
get something, often some domestic gadget or part of a car, working
properly. That's the image to hold in your mind and this helps us to avoid
becoming too cynical.

Task 7.6: Which parts of the curriculum are you tinkering with?

7.6(a) Do you always teach the same thing in *exactly* the same way every
time you teach it?

7.6(b) Should we teach students of science, of nursing, of motor vehicle
maintenance, to exactly the same curriculum in the same ways and
with the same assessment methods as we did five, ten or even
twenty years ago?

We, the writers of this book, believe that the curriculum must develop
continually. All of us will sometimes hanker for a supposed golden age of
education and training lost somewhere in the mists of time but it is
deceptively easy to lose sight of the fact that, in every field, knowledge
has progressed and the demands made on those educated and trained
in that field have changed and intensified. All of this means that the
curriculum must change.

However, remember your answers to Task 7.6 about your own everyday teaching and training. Most of us continually develop our teaching
and training as we learn more about it over the years. The important
thing is to ensure that the curriculum is changed – not to glorify an
individual's or group's political position, but simply to improve the quality
of student learning.

To summarize, therefore, this section has begun a structural survey of
the notion of curriculum by asking you to consider your notion of curriculum and to set it against those of other teachers and trainers and against
ideas from the literature. It has examined some reasons for curriculum

change and concluded that the key criterion of initiating such change should be the improved quality of student learning. The next section will ask you to consider the nature of your own curriculum in more detail.

7.3 *What are the key features of our courses?*

KEY ISSUES

What are the key features of our courses?

How does your course look in relation to others?

What are the key models from the literature on curriculum?

What can curriculum models tell us about our courses?

This section will help us to identify, analyse and review the key characteristics of our courses in terms of purposes, what our students learn and how they learn. To help us to do this critically and rigorously, four curriculum models will be used. This section continues the structural survey of curriculum begun in Section 7.2 and prepares us for a detailed analysis later.

Figure 7.4 presents some teachers' and trainers' statements about how they view the key characteristics of learning in their courses. Notice how each of these statements conveys a sense of purpose and meaning about student learning. Thus, for instance, can you see how Sarah's aims and outcomes (purposes) include students learning the Biology content well enough to achieve GCSE? However, Sarah also says that her students need to begin thinking as scientists, implying that her view of GCSE Biology content is to teach students not simply a set of facts, but also a process of thinking, so that they can gain a better GCSE grade and use scientific thinking in their everyday lives.

Task 7.7: What are the key features of other people's courses?

Choose three of the statements in Figure 7.4 and identify what the teacher/trainer says or implies about:

- the aims and outcomes (purposes) of the course;
- the content of what is being learned;
- the process of that learning.

Figure 7.4 Teachers/trainers talking about their courses

'Our aromatherapy course is about getting students to learn skills, acquire knowledge and to work with clients in a very special way.'

(Suzanne and Nicole)

'My art foundation course tries to help students to assume responsibility for developing and testing their own artistic knowledge, skills and understanding and to take control of their own careers as artists.'

(Mathew)

'My degree courses in different science specialisms all aim to produce practical, all-round scientists who are technically very knowledgeable, but who can also operate very effectively in practical situations and who can communicate and work closely with others.'

(Sam)

'My IT NVQ course gets students to learn how to use a piece of software as required in their workplaces.'

(Angie)

'My first aid course demands students learn basic procedures by heart but that they develop their common sense when dealing with emergency situations.'

(John)

'My bricklaying NVQ course means students need to learn the basic techniques but also need to be able to see how these will lead to a construction . . . see the potential their skills provide.'

(Andy)

'In their initial training on dangerous driving, my police trainees must know their law to the letter but they must also learn how to read a situation and to deal with the public in positive ways.'

(Bob)

'My GCSE biologists must know the Biology syllabus content really well but they must also learn about thinking like scientists.'

(Sarah)

Task 7.8: Key features of your course

Pause before reading on and try to summarize student learning in one of your own courses, or a part of it, in a sentence or so. Make sure you say something about the:

- purposes;
- content;
- process of learning.

Keep your statement handy so that you can refer to it when attempting Task 7.9.

So far in this section we have concentrated on exposing the key features of other teachers' and trainers' courses and comparing them with our own. Let's test our thinking more fully by examining some of the literature on curriculum models. All these ideas can then be used to examine our own courses in more detail.

Interestingly, systematic approaches to developing the curriculum are relatively new, having first appeared in the USA in the 1940s before spreading to the UK in the 1960s. Four curriculum models appear consistently in the curriculum literature and these are summarized below.

The product or objectives model: a focus on *behavioural targets* for learning

This model is interested in the product of a curriculum: just what does it equip a learner to do?

It is closely associated with Ralph Tyler (1971), was one of the earliest curriculum models and has become one of the most influential. Indeed, Tanner and Tanner (1980) argue that it is *the* dominant model of twentieth-century thought about curriculum design. Tyler organizes his model around four fundamental questions which, he claims, must be answered when developing any curriculum:

Figure 7.5 Tyler's model

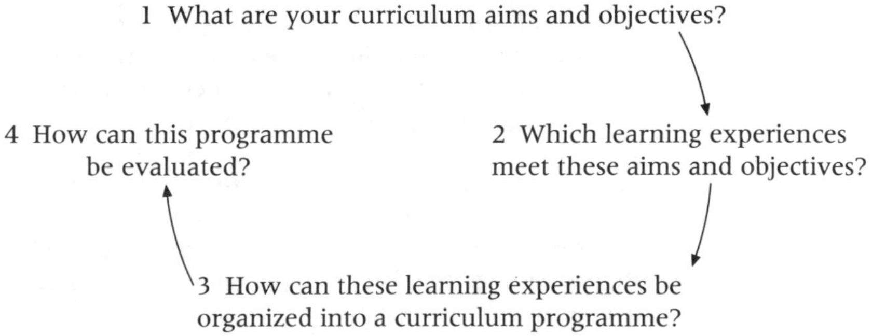

1 What are your curriculum aims and objectives?

4 How can this programme be evaluated?

2 Which learning experiences meet these aims and objectives?

3 How can these learning experiences be organized into a curriculum programme?

Tyler argues that each of these questions requires careful thinking including an element of needs analysis (of both students and others such as employers). Thus, aims and objectives (the purposes of the curriculum) need to rest on the overall purposes (philosophy) of the relevant college, university or training organization, on the view of learning held by the curriculum developers and teachers/trainers, and on the subject matter itself. Once determined, these aims and objectives must specify as clearly and unambiguously as possible what is to be learned. In turn, this will aid the selection and organization of the learning and assessment experiences and the evaluation procedures. All this, of course, links closely into the issues raised in Chapters 3, 5 and 9 of this book.

It is worth noting at this stage that Tyler concentrates on the *how* of curriculum making not the *what* of the curriculum itself (Walker and Soltis 1992). Thus, it is possible to use his four questions to develop courses which will rest on very different notions of learning, teaching and assessment.

However, in practice, this model is widely associated with behaviourist approaches to learning and the curriculum (see Chapter 3). Behavioural objectives are devised which pre-specify measurable learning outcomes. Learning and assessment experiences are then selected and organized to meet these objectives and evaluation takes place to establish how well the course has enabled the specified behaviours to be learned. Students play a largely passive role in all this.

Nevertheless, the Tyler model remains probably the most influential of all and its clarity and simplicity mean that it is an accessible mechanism for curriculum design and development.

The content model: a focus on the *what* of learning

This is an approach to curriculum which is interested in the transmission of existing knowledge to new learners.

The model was developed in the 1950s and 1960s and rests on the work of, among others, Paul Hirst (1974). The emphasis is on the intellectual development of learners. Hirst believes that there are seven or eight forms of knowledge which represent the ways in which people experience and learn about the world. These are mathematics, physical science, knowledge of persons, literature and fine arts, morals, religion and philosophy. The curriculum is, therefore, designed to enable learners to develop their understanding of these areas which usually assume the form of curriculum subjects. Such a curriculum uses objectives but of a broader kind than the purely behavioural type mentioned earlier. The prime aim of the curriculum is the transmission of wisdom – that is, knowledge already developed – often in the form of disciplines or subjects. It is this knowledge that becomes the chief factor influencing any curriculum decisions.

The process model: a focus on the *how* of learning

This is an approach to curriculum which is interested in the processes and procedures of learning so that the learner is able to use and develop the content, not simply receive it passively.

The model was explicitly developed by Lawrence Stenhouse (1975) as a response to the product or objectives model described earlier. The emphasis is on defining content in cognitive terms as concepts and broad-based skills and this, in turn, defines the ways (processes and procedures) through which students need to learn. There is a reliance on teachers being relatively autonomous and possessing a high degree of professional ability since they must have a thorough understanding and judgement of the concepts, principles and criteria inherent in their own subjects (Taylor and Richards 1985).

Thus, teachers need to define the content of their course, define what constitutes a teaching procedure acceptable in subject terms and make clear the standards by which students' work is to be judged (Stenhouse 1975). In this way, Stenhouse sees teachers as being able to plan rationally without using (behavioural) objectives.

The situational model: a focus on the *cultural context* of learning

Dennis Lawton (1983) and Malcolm Skilbeck (1976) are linked to this approach which emphasizes the context in which the curriculum exists.

In short, Lawton sees education as being about the transmission of the key elements of a society's culture to the new generation. His work sees culture as existing in eight subsystems such as economic, technological and aesthetic. The curriculum should then be organized in terms of the knowledge and experiences most appropriate for each subsystem.

Skilbeck sees the culture of the college, university or training organization as a key factor in determining the eventual shape of the curriculum. He advocates what he terms 'situational analysis' – a review of the internal and external issues affecting the organization – as a precursor to using one of the other models. Thus, the situation in which the curriculum will operate becomes a key determinant of its eventual shape.

Task 7.9: What are these curriculum models all about?

Summarize the key aspects of each model (product/objectives, content, process and situational) in your own words. What are their key similarities and differences? Remember to refer back to the statement you made in response to Task 7.8.

At this point it is important to note that all these models are directive in that each lays down a prescription for carrying out the processes of curriculum design and development which allows different views on aims and objectives, content, learning, teaching and assessment to be combined so as to produce a curriculum. As such, theoretical models are useful in helping us to review an existing course or to design a new course since they also carry these proposed solutions to the problems of curriculum design and development.

Let's see if these models can help us in practice by enabling us to identify the key features of our courses. Remember, most of us teach on courses that others have designed even though we usually have some degree of freedom to interpret, sequence and manage the learning experiences of our students. This means that many of our courses are, in practice, a combination of different curriculum models.

For example, take the GCSE Biology course mentioned in Figure 7.4. Sarah went on to describe her course as being 80 per cent content, product and situational and only 20 per cent process. That is, the curriculum seems most focused on getting students following a one-year retake course in an FE college department with a particular way of doing things (situational) to learn biology and to remember it for the examination (content) with the course itself being simply a passport to employment or higher-level courses (product), a view echoed by Sarah's students. The small proportion of process is Sarah trying hard within a tightly defined course and timescale to develop more scientific thinking and behaviour in her students.

In contrast, Andy described his NVQ bricklaying course as being 80 per cent product and 20 per cent content and process. He and his students see the NVQ as mainly a measure of their craft skills and as a means of obtaining and keeping employment. The content and process aspects simply refer to the basic knowledge required by NVQ and the ways in which Andy helps his students to learn.

Finally, Suzanne and Nicole described their aromatherapy course as being one-third product, one-third content and one-third process and situational. This reflects the students' need for qualification in order to practise in many places (product), their need to know what they are doing (content) and the ways in which they must learn to work with clients in an often quite intimate fashion (process), something both Suzanne and Nicole felt to be particularly important in their profession (situational).

Task 7.10: Your course and the four models

Consider a course you teach in relation to the four curriculum models. Make a rough judgement about which of the models features in your course and in what proportions. What are the reasons for your answer?

There is a key lesson in all of this regarding how to treat theoretical models: use them not as a 'quick fix' but as tools to analyse the purpose, the selection and organization of learning and assessment activities and evaluation procedures.

Most teachers and trainers in PCE find that their courses are a particular combination of product, content, process and situation. Each course will have its own points of emphasis. Take the Certificate of Education itself, for instance. It has a clear product emphasis (a trained teacher/trainer with a national qualification), a content dimension (the knowledge and understanding required of a fully trained professional) and process and situational aspects (the ways in which you learn and gain the qualification and the context in which the qualification is provided). While each of the four models seems to claim that it presents the correct way to develop a curriculum, in reality we need to balance a wide range of factors in order to arrive at a workable curriculum that can operate in practical situations. Curriculum models can, however, help us to be more thoughtful and professional in this process.

One further point is worth making. Although four models have been outlined and examined in this section, many of us have found that, in practice, we end up using the set of four questions posed by Tyler (1971) (see p. 169). This is certainly not because we are all behavioural objectives enthusiasts but because the questions provide a straightforward framework for developing our courses. Indeed, many of our own students have pointed out that, in essence, the other models eventually arrive at a similar set of questions. The key thing is to ensure that, before you begin the curriculum development process you have a clear idea about how you view learning and your subject matter. Then, Tyler's questions can help you build a practical curriculum.

To summarize, this section has continued the structural survey of curriculum by asking you to identify the purposes, content, process and context of your courses in relation to similar statements from other teachers and trainers. It has presented and examined four curriculum models and identified their key characteristics. You have set your own courses against the four models in order to clarify the precise nature of your courses. Finally, the section has provided advice on the use of theoretical models and has concluded that, in practice, all our courses contain elements of all the models, and it is the proportions that expose the differences. Bearing this in mind, Tyler's questions might be a useful framework provided we have already thought about our positions on learning and subject matter.

Having identified the key characteristics of our courses, the next section will ask why our courses possess these characteristics and investigate the assumptions, values and purposes that underpin them.

7.4 What ideologies (values, assumptions and purposes) underpin our courses?

KEY ISSUES

Why are courses organized so differently?

Why are there so many different curriculum models?

Should there be this variety in both theory and practice?

The previous section used practical and theoretical methods to help us to begin a review of our courses but it also showed the variety in curriculum theory (four different models) and practice – just look at the different responses of those teachers and trainers talking about their courses in Figure 7.4. This section asks why this variety exists, if it is necessary and, if so, why it is so important.

The 1980s saw the start of a concerted effort by government to reduce curriculum variety (see Chapter 1), and in particular since 1988 the compulsory education sector has seen the continuing evolution of the National Curriculum in an attempt to establish national benchmarks and to raise standards. Meanwhile post-compulsory education and training has seen, among other changes, the development of NVQs to bring national standards to vocational training, and the complete reorganization of both the nurse and police training curricula to produce nurses and police officers with the knowledge, skills and abilities required for their rapidly changing roles in society. More recently, there has been the introduction of GNVQ (a supposed mix of academic education and vocational training) and changes to A levels to reduce the proliferation of syllabuses and to ensure the maintenance of standards. The early years of the twenty-first century might well see wholesale changes to A level and GNVQ leading to a baccalaureate style of provision, to prevent excess specialization and to promote breadth with rigour, and more standardization across first degree courses to guarantee the quality of first degrees across all universities.

However, even if the formal curriculum, the printed syllabus or specification is standardized, does that mean the curriculum in practice – as taught by teachers/trainers and experienced by learners – is standardized?

Task 7.11: Same course, same learning experience?

7.11(a) When you were at school, did all the teachers of the same subject, say maths, teach in the same way? Explain your answer.

7.11(b) In your own area of teaching/training, does every teacher/trainer work in an identical way? Explain your answer.

7.11(c) Do you think that the following groups of learners have identical learning experiences? Explain your answers.

- all the first-year economics degree students in a university;
- all NVQ Level 3 beauty therapy trainees in college or a workplace;
- all police probationary constables in a training centre.

So, assuming that your answers point towards some variation, however much the formal curriculum is standardized, the question remains as to why this variation exists. And we still haven't answered the question about variation existing between the theoretical models and between curricula. For instance, why is NVQ different from the National Curriculum which is different from A level? And why has GNVQ undergone successive changes since being introduced in 1992?

In short, the answer is that every curriculum represents a set of fundamental beliefs, assumptions and values, collectively termed 'ideologies', about the nature of education and training. As Barnes (1982: 60) says:

> No curriculum planning is neutral: every curriculum is imbued with values. These values embody a view of the kind of people we wish our pupils to become . . . and of the kind of society that such people could live in . . . As Eisner (1969) once wrote when discussing the idea of neutral curriculum planning, under the rug of technique, there lies an image of man.

We can cluster these beliefs about education and training into groups and call these 'educational ideologies' – that is, systems of meanings about education. In order to review and develop our own courses as teachers/trainers, we need to be able to identify these ideologies and hold our own considered position about them.

This is important because these ideologies include assumptions about learning, teaching, the nature of subject knowledge and about how education and training are linked to the wider economic, political, moral and social circumstances of the time. All this sets the context for making decisions about what to teach, how students should learn and how such learning should be assessed.

So, just what are these ideologies and how do they relate to education and training? Scrimshaw (1983) identifies five major educational ideologies which together represent over 2000 years of thinking about the nature and meaning of education and training. They are now briefly described.

Classical humanism: maintaining a stable society by transmitting society's cultural heritage to students

Over 2000 years ago in ancient Greece, Plato, in the *Meno* (1956), developed a view of education as being a way of producing a just and harmonious society made up of rational and reflective individuals. His notions of just and harmonious were tied to an hierarchical society with the role of education being to train people to take up their proper roles. Thus, people at different levels in the hierarchy would require different curricula with only the rulers needing a full education in philosophy and the mathematical sciences because they were the only people who would need to develop wisdom.

Interestingly, around 1000 years later, St Augustine devised a very similar proposal. He wanted a general education consisting of seven liberal arts to be provided to most pupils while a select few were to be given studies in philosophy and theology, ready to command a society dominated by the Christian Church.

Liberal humanism: the use of the intellectual disciplines in developing individuals and, thus, a fairer and more equal society

In the eighteenth century as, post-Renaissance, the thinkers of the Enlightenment period attempted to envisage a society beyond that controlled by hereditary monarchs, Rousseau (see Boyd 1956) advocated a view of society which assumed people to be naturally good but too often corrupted by their social environments.

For Rousseau, education was about providing structure, order and discipline to help learners develop into morally mature individuals. The curriculum would be developmental, take great account of individual differences and begin with everyday situations before moving on to a systematic study of the essential disciplines of literature, history, science, mathematics etc. (Taylor and Richards 1985). All this would, argued Rousseau, produce free thinking, responsible individuals able to play their full part in a free and democratic society.

Progressivism: meeting individuals' needs and aspirations so as to support their personal growth and strengthen a democratic society

In the early twentieth century in the USA, Dewey (1915) developed an approach which saw both the above ideologies as problematic. He saw classical humanism as too teacher-centred, too concerned with existing knowledge and with fitting people into an existing society. Liberal humanism, on the other hand, he considered too student-centred, ignoring the importance of the social contexts of learning and development. So, he developed a middle way, between these two.

This involved Dewey's own vision of democracy as the best way for people in a society to live together and for individuals to grow and develop. He wanted schools that replicated democracy in an 'embryonic social community' in which students were encouraged to cooperate and work together and learn from each other as well as from their teachers (Walker and Soltis 1992). Education was to extend people's powers and possibilities as human beings. The curriculum would be based around active problem-solving in a variety of social contexts and be constructed of topics which interested and challenged students (learning from experience) with the aim that people would learn how to think for themselves, make decisions, cooperate and participate as makers of a democratic society.

Instrumentalism: a curriculum delivering a specific product such as the development of a skilled workforce

This ideology has become an increasingly important element in UK government policy since the Great Debate was initiated in 1976 and, with the election of the Labour government in 1997, shows every sign of remaining at the heart of government policy.

Instrumentalism as it operates in the UK at the turn of the twentieth century, sees a highly educated workforce as essential in meeting growing international competition and values high levels of numeracy and literacy, subject areas covering aspects of science and technology and anything else seen as relevant to achieving this goal. The instrumental curriculum sees knowledge in factual terms and is clearly teacher/trainer led. Thus, through instrumentalist education and training, students are preparing themselves for their roles in the workplace and in society as a whole.

Reconstructionism: education to change society

In stark contrast to the other ideologies, reconstructionism sees education as the means of moving society in a particular direction; in effect, as a tool of the state. In many developing countries, some degree of reconstructionism is, perhaps, necessary, as they seek to raise the living standards of their populations through a largely product-oriented curriculum.

However, totalitarian governments have always used education as a means of getting people to serve the interests of those in power and there are numerous past examples including Nazi Germany, the Soviet Union and, at the time of writing, China, where the purpose of education is described in Taylor and Richards (1985: 21) as being: 'to serve the ends of proletarian politics, not the pursuit of individual goals and aspirations'. Interestingly, in the late 1990s, China is several years into a policy of using education as part of its attempt to move towards a more open, market-based economy while maintaining the political and social status quo. Clearly, time will tell if this will be successful.

Task 7.12: What are these five ideologies all about?

Summarize the key aspects of each educational ideology by commenting on the following:

• what is the historical origin of the ideology?
• how does it view the role of education and training?
• what kind of curriculum is advocated?
• what is the value given to individual learners?

Most courses in post-compulsory education and training are influenced fairly clearly in their make-up by an ideology even if this is applied inconsistently, mixed with another and applied without universal agreement.

Task 7.13: Spot the ideology

Look at a course you teach and see if you can link it to a particular ideology. Explain your responses. Or, looking at the following courses, which ideology(ies) would you associate with any three of them? Explain your responses.

- NVQ
- Nurse training
- A levels
- AE
- MBA
- Police training
- GNVQ
- University degrees
- Numberpower

Having arrived at your responses to Tasks 7.12 and 7.13, consider one further issue. Are these fundamental assumptions, values and beliefs which underpin every course made explicit to teacher/trainers and learners? Is it simply assumed either that these are matters too obvious to be missed or that everyone else agrees and, therefore, no mention is necessary? What does your course documentation say about any of this? It is the unspoken and, all too often, the non-debated nature of ideologies in education that can cause difficulties for everyone.

In conclusion, therefore, this section has tackled the question as to why courses seem to vary so much both in theory and in practice. In essence, it is because course developers and those commissioning courses have their own assumptions, beliefs and values about the nature and purpose of education and training and these ideologies affect course design. In an age when courses seem likely to become more, rather than less, standardized, variation will still occur because teachers/trainers have their own ideologies and this will affect the ways they teach and train their students.

In terms of helping us with our own work, two issues need mentioning. First, as we review and develop our own courses, we must be explicit about our ideologies so that our colleagues, and other teachers/trainers and students will understand our intentions. Second, when we come to use other people's courses, we need to be able to identify the ideological underpinnings in order to arrive at how we will operate the course in practice.

7.5 *Where do you stand so far?*

KEY ISSUES

What is your working definition of curriculum?

How can the four curriculum models be of help?

Where do you stand in terms of educational ideology?

The purpose of this section is to provide an opportunity for us to pause a moment so as to review and record where we have got to in thinking about the theory and practice of curriculum matters. On the basis of this, we can then move forward to plan and develop a new, or revised, curriculum.

Task 7.14: Reporting on your review of curriculum

7.14(a) What is your definition of curriculum?

7.14(b) Why should the curriculum always be developing?

7.14(c) Use the curriculum models to help analyse a course you teach on. What mixture of product, content, process and situation is it?

7.14(d) What educational ideology do you feel most comfortable with? Why?

7.14(e) What ideology lies behind a course you teach on? If it's different from your response to 7.14(d), does this raise any practical issues?

As practising teachers/trainers, this chapter has presented you with opportunities to consider your own work and that of other teachers/trainers. In order to help you, some of the theoretical work on curriculum has been introduced so that you can become more critical and thoughtful. However, have you noticed the different ways we can treat curriculum theory? The curriculum models are there to aid review and development and they provide ways of sorting out curriculum matters. So, in practice, our own courses often represent a particular combination of models.

Ideologies, however, are different. They represent our fundamental beliefs about the nature and purpose of a curriculum. Although some overlap of ideas is natural, we can only really embed the ideas of *one* ideology in any curriculum.

So, having completed our structural survey of the curriculum, it's time to start planning and building. All this now means we can move on to Chapter 8 where we will begin to design and develop a new or revised curriculum, establish thorough evaluation mechanisms and be able to present and justify our new or revised course to others.

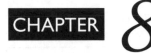

COURSE DESIGN, DEVELOPMENT AND EVALUATION

8.1 *What is Chapter 8 about?*

Given the increasing degree of central control over courses evident in recent years, we might be forgiven for assuming that, as teachers and trainers, we have little or no role to play in course design and development. This is far from true.

Even highly prescribed courses such as NVQ, GNVQ and A level, or occupation-specific training programmes such as those for police officers or nurses still leave us, working as individuals or as part of a team, relatively free to interpret, sequence, resource and emphasize the various course elements in our own way, drawing on our own professional judgement to decide what will maximize opportunities for our students to learn. In this way we are able to design and develop the curriculum. This is a vital element in our work as teachers and trainers. Indeed, in examining curriculum design and development in some detail, this chapter views it as something which contributes to the overall aim of the book – to develop teachers' and trainers' professional abilities and to nourish their critical awareness.

This chapter focuses on the ways that we, as teachers and trainers structure and organize students' learning. It challenges readers to examine the very courses they teach. Sections 8.2 and 8.3 ask how a curriculum might be designed and developed, and how its effectiveness can be evaluated and judged. Section 8.4 examines how such new developments can be presented to colleges and training organizations so that they might be put into operation.

8.2   *Designing and developing your course*

> KEY ISSUES
>
> How can we develop or revise a course?
>
> What is the role of ideology and curriculum models?
>
> How can we identify what's needed in the new or revised course?
>
> How can we specify course purposes?
>
> How can we sequence and organize course content into learning and assessment experiences?

Sooner or later, as teachers or trainers, we all need to handle aspects of course design and development. For instance, starting a new job and planning our teaching, deciding how we will put into practice a current syllabus or NVQ/GNVQ specification by turning it into a practical course, revising a course that has been running for a while, or setting up a new course from scratch are all tasks that we need to be able to carry out professionally. The question is, how?

This section will provide some practical answers based on a straightforward model derived from the theoretical and practical work described in Chapter 7. It makes no claims for being anything more than a practical framework by setting out a sequence of six stages for curriculum developers to follow, shown in Figure 8.1.

Figure 8.1 A model for curriculum design and development

Stage 1	Select a manageable course development task (it's got to be practical!)
Stage 2	Consider the ideological basis for the course, to identify its key values, beliefs and assumptions
Stage 3	Conduct a needs analysis: if favourable, continue development work to ensure the proposed course really is worthwhile and practical
Stage 4	Develop statements of purpose (aims and objectives) to set clear intentions and outcomes in the light of the above
Stage 5	Specify content and sequence, then organize appropriate learning and assessment experiences, to enable learners to achieve the intentions and purposes
Stage 6	Establish appropriate evaluation and feedback procedures, to review and improve the effectiveness of the course for learners

This section will cover Stages 1 to 5. That is, it will take you from identifying a manageable course development task through to selecting content and designing a full scheme of work. The final stage, that of course evaluation and feedback, will be tackled in the next section. Evaluation is given its own section because its importance is often underestimated, with the result that it is simply tacked on at the end of a course, seemingly as a bit of an afterthought.

Stage 1: Select a manageable course development task

The starting point is defining the kind of course that is needed – something that might be easier said than done! However, in order for you to gain the maximum benefit from the remainder of this chapter, you should have a curriculum development task to work on. Examples of courses developed by Certificate of Education students in recent years are shown in Figure 8.2. Whatever you choose to focus on, try to make sure it's relevant to your work as a teacher/trainer and that it's something manageable.

Figure 8.2 Examples of courses developed by Certificate of Education students

---

- Driving instructor training
- Brass band music for beginners
- Introductory sculpture
- Preparing for life at university
- Equal opportunities for special constables
- Outreach course for deprived youngsters
- Induction for early years workers
- NVQ IT training
- Bricklaying for DIYers
- Students with special needs: a course for FE teachers
- How to have a good time and stay healthy
- LGV driver training
- Introductory reflexology

- Conflict management
- Introduction to a new IT system
- Minibus driver training
- Art and group therapy
- Various A-level courses
- BA/BSc modules and units
- French for shopworkers
- NVQ customer care
- Health and safety at work
- Presentation skills
- Police promotion skills
- European art summer school
- Bereavement care for nurses
- Women's health and body care
- GNVQ business units
- C&G gardening
- Suturing for nurses
- GNVQ health and social care

Task 8.1: What curriculum to develop?

Select a course (or a part of it) you teach that you need to revise, or identify a syllabus, specification or subject you would like to teach (or that your organization has decided you should teach) but which needs developing into a practical course.

Once you have identified your curriculum development task, the next question for you to address is just what kind of course do you want it to be?

Stage 2: Consider the ideological basis for the course

Task 8.2: What kind of course and why?

Remember Chapter 7 and your own educational ideology that it helped you to define.

8.2(a) What educational ideology (fundamental values, beliefs and assumptions) will you bring to the job of course design development?

8.2(b) If you are revising an existing course, or developing a course from a pre-set syllabus or specification, what seems to be its underlying ideology?

8.2(c) If your answers to 8.2(a) and (b) are different, can you balance the two? Explain how.

Your responses to Task 8.2 will act as a framework around which you can begin to develop your course. However, now that you have clarified the kind of course you want to develop, what needs must the course meet, and how are you to identify these, especially students' learning needs?

Stage 3: Conduct a needs analysis

What needs must this course meet? Perhaps this is better rephrased to read *whose* needs? Quite naturally, this will depend on a whole range of factors including you, any of your colleagues who might be involved, the organization within which you are working, those who might use the course to make judgements (such as employers, colleges, universities) and, most important of all, the learners themselves.

Task 8.3: Whose needs and why?

List those with needs to be taken account of in planning your course. Why do you have to take their needs into account?

Figure 8.3 Questions for a needs analysis

1 What are your organization's criteria for numbers, costs, accommodation, staffing and resources?
2 Is there any demand for the course?
3 How long is the demand estimated to last?
4 Are there any similar courses running in the area? If so, will there be sufficient demand for all to run?
5 What is the estimated size of the potential student population?
6 What would a profile of the prospective students show?
7 Will the course appear in league tables?
8 What costs will the course incur?
9 Will the course attract any funding?
10 For those courses attracting fee paying students, what price will prospective students be willing to pay?
11 What does the assessment and evaluation data from previous cohorts contain?
12 How was any previous needs analysis carried out? What information does it contain?
13 Can other staff who have been involved provide you with any additional information?
14 Will your course meet the organization's criteria?

So, given these needs must be met, how are you to identify and analyse them? Just what is a 'needs analysis'? In short, it involves the collection and analysis of information from all those who will be involved and affected by the proposed course so that the planning stage can take account of as wide a range of needs as is practicable.

Obviously, this requires careful handling because every course demands a different level of needs analysis. For instance, if you are revising an existing course you should already have at least some basic information about needs which might simply need reviewing and extending in places. If, on the other hand, you are developing a brand new curriculum then a much more detailed needs analysis will be required before you make any further progress. Figure 8.3 provides a set of suggested questions, the answers to which would result in a full needs analysis report. If you are revising a course, choose whichever seem most appropriate.

Having identified the kind of needs analysis you intend to carry out, you have then to decide how this information will be obtained. Figure 8.4 provides some suggestions. However, don't set up complicated surveys involving large numbers of people or feel obliged to cost everything to the last penny unless you are involved in a really large-scale development. Use your organization's support staff to help (for example, if a technical costing is required) and be realistic. It's a matter of generating sufficient information on the basis of which you, your colleagues and your organization might make a professional judgement.

Figure 8.4 Possible strategies for needs analysis data collection

- *Meeting the organization's criteria* – liaise with others in the organization to clarify criteria and report back with information.
- *Judging demand size and longevity* – monitor any feeder routes for prospective students, e.g. conduct surveys of schools, employers, colleges, universities.
- *Identifying the competition* – survey other providers.
- *Profiling prospective students* – once you have identified feeder routes, survey these prospective students to identify their particular needs.
- *Costing* – accurate estimated costs of staffing, accommodation, resources, food/drink, administration, examination etc. as appropriate.
- *Funding* – checks with organizations such as FEFC, HEFCE, TEC (Training and Enterprise Council), LEAs (Local education authorities), NHS (National Health Service) trusts, police forces, etc. as appropriate.
- *Pricing* – survey of prospective students and of competition prices.
- *Learning from previous experience* – use existing assessment and evaluation data; liaise with other staff.

Task 8.4: Conducting a needs analysis

8.4(a) Using Figures 8.3 and 8.4, conduct a needs analysis for your proposed course.

8.4(b) Summarize your findings in a report which will form part of your curriculum development documentation.

Having conducted and reported on the needs analysis, and assuming we are going ahead, the next stage is to specify or review the purposes of the course, often presented as aims and objectives.

Stage 4: Develop statements of purpose (aims and objectives)

Course purposes are shaped by two key things. First, the ideology underpinning the course (already specified in Task 8.2). Second, the curriculum model, or combination of models, representing the key features of the intended course. For example, a progressive ideology and process curriculum model would lead to aims and objectives emphasizing individual learner development and growth whereas classical humanism and a product curriculum would aim for learners gaining specified kinds and quantities of knowledge in order to fulfil specified roles in society.

Task 8.5: Factors affecting course purposes

Consider what model or combination of curriculum models will best support the course you are developing. Take into account your own preferences and, if relevant, the emphasis apparent in the syllabus of specification.

There is another dimension to stating purposes. You may recall that Chapter 3 introduced several different approaches to learning which would have a clear effect on aims, which are broad statements of purpose, and, in particular, objectives, which are much more specific course or lesson targets and learning outcomes. For example, an expressly behavioural perspective on learning will lead to objectives very different to those generated from a purely cognitive approach. Figure 8.5, adapted from Cohen and Manion (1989: 32–41) presents some guidance on two different types of objective.

Figure 8.5 Defining, writing and using two types of objective

Key characteristics of behavioural objectives
- specify who is to perform the desired behaviour;
- specify this behaviour clearly and unambiguously;
- specify the conditions for the behaviour to be demonstrated;
- specify the standard used to determine success or failure.

Using behavioural objectives
- requires great care because it defines learning in one particular way (behaviourally);
- requires teachers/trainers to be sure this is appropriate for the course and the intended learning;
- is better not done unless these conditions are met.

Key characteristics of non-behavioural objectives
- may be more flexible and open-ended;
- still need expressing simply and linking to learning experiences;
- allow for broader notions of learning to be used, not just behaviour.

When to use each type of objective
- Behavioural objectives might well be most effective when the subject matter and intended learning is skill-based and can be demonstrated easily, or where overt writing or speaking can demonstrate appropriate levels of learning, or where learners need small, behavioural stages brought into the subject matter to provide clear, attainable targets.
- Non-behavioural objectives might be best used when the intended learning is more complex or less specific, is developmental and almost impossible to view in terms of behaviour without reducing the learning to an absurd level.

Source: Cohen and Manion 1989.

Task 8.6 provides some examples of behavioural and non-behavioural objectives from Certificate of Education students' course development work.

Task 8.6: Examples of course objectives

From the list below, identify which objectives are behavioural and which are non-behavioural, and think about why.

The student will be able to:

• demonstrate how to grip the (golf) club correctly;
• demonstrate how to place a casualty into the recovery position;
• increase their understanding of the theories of loss and bereavement;
• appreciate the importance of taking responsibility for their own health;
• open a file, input data, save the data and exit from a database program;
• identify and meet necessary health and safety regulations;
• feel more confident about using the specialist equipment;
• understand the thinking behind a theoretical model in economics;
• become a more reflective and critical professional;
• drive a minibus to Driving Standards Agency standards.

Having identified the main issues involved in expressing the purposes of a course through aims and objectives, there are two further points to make. First, when you come to write your course aims and objectives, keep them to the minimum necessary to specify the course intentions fully. Second, don't be afraid to mix behavioural and non-behavioural objectives provided you make it clear that you are doing this deliberately.

For example, in an NVQ healthcare assistants' course, your students will certainly need to meet the performance criteria which are, as with all NVQs, behavioural objectives and learning outcomes. However, you might also want to include in your practical operation of the course some more broadly based, non-behavioural objectives to cover the less obvious but very important aspects of working with patients on a busy ward. So, if your course intends learning of different kinds to take place, the objectives must recognize this. Just be honest and show you have been thoughtful about it.

All this means that we have reached the next stage, that of identifying and sequencing appropriate teaching/training and assessment experiences for our prospective students.

Stage 5: Specify content and sequence, then organize appropriate learning and assessment experiences

For many of us, these are the tasks we immediately associate with the notion of course development. Indeed, we might well relish the work because it involves us in working out what we consider to be the programme through which students can learn our specialist subject most effectively.

However, it is not too long before a number of key questions arise. How is content chosen, or rejected? What makes for a correct sequence? How are learning and assessment experiences linked to all this? Is a detailed plan required for each session or will a scheme of work suffice? Just what level of detail is required at this stage in the development of a new or revised course? The remainder of this section will provide some practical answers to these questions.

How is content chosen? In many cases course content is already specified by a syllabus or, in the case of NVQ, may be identified in relation to the course specification. In other cases, teachers/trainers might have a much freer choice. However, don't forget our earlier work in this chapter which indicated that, however tightly specified the course content might be, and no matter how well-known and commonly covered it is, individual teachers/trainers will always provide their students with (however slightly) different experiences. We can take nothing for granted here. All of us need to consider the content we teach and the basis on which we have chosen it.

Task 8.7: Thinking about content and sequence

Choose one of the following contexts:

1 Ben, a 9-month-old baby, is with you in his bedroom playing. Please get him bathed and changed etc. ready to go to sleep.
2 Jo, a learner driver, is going along a residential road at 25m.p.h. and needs to turn the car around and drive back the way she has come. What does she need to do?

8.7(a) Using one of the above contexts what, in your opinion, is the best practice sequence in which the activity should be carried out?

8.7(b) What content do learner parents or drivers need to understand in order for them to achieve the objective of a (near) perfect performance?

Figure 8.6 presents two sets of responses from Certificate of Education students to the first context in Task 8.7, bathing a baby. Note the differences. Is one of the sequences better? Why? What about the content involved? Would either or both sets of responses achieve the objective?

Group A explained that their objective was to achieve the bathing of the baby and that safety, hygiene and careful handling were the prime objectives and content to be used. In contrast, Group B stated that, for them, bathtime was an important element in the baby's routine, in elementary learning about water and hygiene, but that it can be fun too and an aid in developing the child's relationship with its parent(s) and, thus, its overall development. It was also seen by one student as having

Figure 8.6 How to bathe a baby?

Group A response	*Group B response*
1 Warm baby clothes	1 Make sure baby is happily and safely playing in bedroom
2 Warm towel	
3 Run bath	2 Warm clothes, run water, test, put in bath toys and bubbles
4 Take baby to bathroom	
5 Test water temperature	3 Bring in baby, start tape of bathtime songs and sing along
6 Undress baby and remove nappy	
	4 Remove soiled nappy and clean baby as needed while singing
7 Place baby carefully in bath	
8 Wash carefully and hygienically	5 Place baby gently in bath, reassure using toys and music
9 Remove baby from bath carefully	6 Wash baby carefully, using different cloth for face, still singing and playing
10 Wrap baby in towel and dry	
11 Use cream etc. and put on fresh nappy	7 Carry on playing etc. as seems best
12 Take baby to bedroom	8 Gently remove baby from bath and wrap in warm towel
13 Dress baby	
14 Lie baby safely in cot	9 Dry baby carefully and apply cream/powder as appropriate
	10 Dress baby and begin playing going to bed game
	11 Turn off music, take baby to bedroom and lay him in cot
	12 Play going to sleep game, read, play music etc. as appropriate
	13 Bring game to an end and settle baby safely down to sleep
	14 Clean and tidy bathroom

been an enjoyable time for the parent too! In other words, ideologically and in terms of curriculum models, these groups had very different starting points which led, in turn, to different content and, to a lesser extent in this example, differences in sequence.

Task 8.8: Reviewing your sequence and content

Look back at your response to Task 8.7. How did you define the objective? Which ideology and curriculum model(s) influenced your sequence and content? Would you want to revise your response at all?

In order to identify the appropriate content and sequence for your proposed course, it is important to take account of two key factors. First, the syllabus or specification and its associated content, ideology and model(s). Second, your own educational ideology and what seems to you to be the most appropriate curriculum model(s), as expressed in your aims and objectives. You must strike a balance between the course as laid out and your own ideas if your content and sequence are to enable the students to achieve your aims and objectives.

Assuming you were about to teach parents to bathe their babies, what kinds of learning and assessment experiences would you use to help them learn? Again, the answer is linked to the balance struck between the course and your own ideas. Thus, to caricature Group A's position, they might be tempted to hire an expert to run a series of lectures entitled 'How to bathe a baby: the way to infant hygiene and safety', with slides, data on water temperature and accidents to babies in bathrooms. Worksheets might be used to enable learning facts and procedures by rote, there would be practice sessions with dolls and participants' performance might be assessed through observation of the practice and some written tests.

Being equally unfair to Group B, on the other hand, they might run a series of workshops entitled 'Hygiene and hugs: making bathtime an enriching experience for all – an holistic perspective'. These would involve parents, a health visitor and a child psychologist working with a facilitator who would start from everyone's own experiences. Through discussion, inputs and home visits by the professionals, some reflection (a reflective log?) and the use of students' own children (and bathrooms!) everything would be brought together. Assessment would be informal and based on participants' contributions, involvement and evidence of their reflection.

Thus, your selection of learning and assessment experiences will emerge directly from all your previous work on developing the course. Assessment was handled fully in Chapter 6. It is mentioned here simply to emphasize its role in providing information to all those involved about what has and has not been learned.

One further question remains with regard to selecting content, sequence and learning and assessment experiences. As part of the process of course development or revision, is every session to be planned in detail? At this stage, the simple answer is no, unless what is being planned is a short event of some kind, say a one-day introduction to a new IT program. In this case, the full day's programme, resources and materials would be required.

In other cases, where longer and more involved courses are under development, what's needed is an outline scheme of work for the course and, usually, one short session (about an hour) which is planned and resourced to provide an indication of quality. As an illustration, Table 8.1 provides an example of part of a scheme of work.

Table 8.1 An example of a scheme of work from a curriculum development proposal

GNVQ Advanced Business scheme of work for Elements 1.1, 3.1, 3.3: 'Marketing and Effects of Supply and Demand on Business' (1996)

Session	Performance Criteria (PC)	IT key skill	Content	Methods	Resource	Outcome	Assessment
1	PC 1.1.1 PC 3.1.1		Introduction to marketing principles	Lecture, discussion, brainstorm	Students' ideas, Teacher input, OHPs	Initial thinking and ideas	Informal through class discussion
2	PC 3.1.2		Case study of a marketing function (traditional)	Individuals summarize main points from case study	GNVQ advanced textbook	Recognize main points in a sales and marketing plan and where they fit in	Informal through viewing individual findings, formal via individual reports
3	PC 3.3.3		Launching a new product onto the market	Guest speaker (medical company sales rep)	Speaker's handout on what to include in plan	Commercial company's perspective on a real problem	Written notes by each student
4	PC 3.1.3		The marketing mix	Video and discussion	Video	Theoretical base	
5	PC 3.1.4 PC 3.1.3 PC 3.3.4		Analysing marketing activities	Visit to blood transfusion centre and presentation by manager	Video, OHP, speaker's ideas and information package	Assignment set and budget limits set giving a real task and consultancy feel to work	
6	Evidence indicators for not-for-profit organizations in 3.1 and 3.3	Key IT PC 3.1.1 PC 3.2.1	Pooling of ideas	Ideas from all students noted	Flip chart and ideas	Central pool of ideas for all students to access	Informal through student discussion
7		PC 3.1.2 PC 3.1.5 PC 3.1.4 PC 3.3.3	Initial work on plan	Individual study and research, formal review of progress with teacher	Books, computers, information packs, students' and teachers' ideas/notes, central pool of ideas	Progress on sales and marketing plan, basic groundwork and initial drafting	Informal through teacher and student discussion
8	PC 3.1 PC 1.2 PC 3.3	PC 3.2.3 PC 3.3.7 PC 3.3.1 PC 3.3.6	Prepare presentation	Individual preparation on aspects of plan	Flip chart, computer, book, notes	Structure for presentation arrived at	
9			Presentation given and assignment submitted	Individuals present aspects of work to class	Flip charts, OHPS, assignments	Sharing ideas, constructive evaluation of others' ideas	Completed assignment and student presentations

Source: Dunnill *et al.* 1995: 135.

Task 8.9: Selecting and sequencing content and deciding on learning and assessment experiences

Begin working on an outline scheme of work for your proposed course which will show how you intend students to achieve the aims and objectives specified earlier. Select and sequence your course content and, given practical limits to time and resources, decide on the kinds of learning and assessment experiences which will be most appropriate. Present them using the exemplar scheme of work layout in Table 8.1 or use one of your own.

To summarize, this section has presented you with the challenge of developing or revising your own course. On the basis of the work presented in previous sections a six stage model for course design and development has been used and this section has taken you through five of these stages, to a point where your course is beginning to take practical shape. The importance of the definitions, ideologies and curriculum models discussed in Chapter 7 has been stressed as a means of ensuring continuity and coherence of learning in your new course. The next section will address the final stage of course development, that of devising effective and appropriate evaluation and feedback procedures.

8.3 *Evaluating your course*

KEY ISSUES

What is evaluation?

Why evaluate? For what purpose and for whom?

What are you going to evaluate?

How and when will you evaluate?

How can you ensure evaluation data feeds back into your course planning cycle?

Just as you thought you were safe! Having put time and effort into the processes of reviewing your existing course, then developing a new course or revising an existing one, you assumed that was that. A job well done. The course is ready to run and you're, rightly, proud of your work. But no! Here is one last stage to work your way through. Surely, you groan, evaluation is just about filling in a form (sometimes) at the end of a course and little or nothing being done afterwards?

So, just what is evaluation and why is it so important? Before going further, consider your responses to Task 8.10.

Task 8.10: Evaluation: your starting point

8.10(a) How regularly does evaluation take place?

8.10(b) How appropriate and user-friendly are your evaluation methods?

8.10(c) Do you let people use their own words at all?

8.10(d) Do you evaluate in ways other than end-of-course forms?

8.10(e) Do you evaluate against practically-described learning purposes?

8.10(f) Do you discuss the results internally, externally, never?

8.10(g) Does anyone else get to know of the results?

8.10(h) Do you ever change anything afterwards?

Evaluation is all about finding out if our new course is working properly. In general, therefore, it involves generating data through a process of inquiry and then, on the basis of this, making judgements about the strengths and weaknesses and the overall effectiveness of the course and making decisions about how to improve it further. As Cronbach (1980: 14) says: '. . . the history of social reform . . . is littered with examples of large-scale and costly catastrophes as well as more modest mistakes . . . evaluation offers to certify that a programme will live up to its advertising'.

There are people who use the words 'evaluation' and 'assessment' as if they were the same thing. Be careful. Assessment refers to information and judgements about individual students' learning. Evaluation is about gaining information and judgements about course effectiveness.

It is important to see if our development work has succeeded and that our new course is meeting its aims and objectives. But there are others who are interested in our work and evaluation has to meet their needs too. So just who are these others?

Earlier sections of this chapter listed several groups who will be interested. As well as the course developers these include the students, the teachers/trainers, others such as managers in our organization together with employers, colleges and universities. We might well add funders, as many funding organizations such as the TECs, organizations within the NHS or the police service, charitable trusts, research sponsors and private companies will insist on evaluation as part of their funding criteria. Finally, in a wider national and global sense, given the increasing climate of accountability, the community in general is often involved and interested in evaluation findings.

All this means that evaluation can become very complicated, an issue we will deal with later in this section. However, in general, it means that any evaluation must specify its intended audience and then ensure it covers all their interests and not simply those of the course developer(s).

Task 8.11: Evaluation: what, why and for whom?

8.11(a) Provide a definition of evaluation and say why it is not assessment.

8.11(b) Why is evaluation an important part of course development?

8.11(c) For your course, who might be interested in an evaluation and why?

Having established the need for an evaluation, what is going to be evaluated? Partly, as was argued in Chapter 7, this will depend on the course ideology and curriculum model(s) – that is, the kind of curriculum you have developed. However, you must also be clear about the main purpose of your evaluation. Is it to help course improvement, to establish its impact and outcomes or some combination of the two? And how much time and money is available, if any? Whatever you decide, ensure you are undertaking something which is practical. Considering these questions will help you to identify what you want to evaluate.

Even when you know the course well there may still be difficulties in deciding what to evaluate, or, as is often the case, what to leave out of an evaluation. Figure 8.7 presents two approaches to this question generated

Figure 8.7 Deciding what to evaluate: two approaches

Group A listed the main things that seem to happen in the course, e.g.:

- are aims and objectives being achieved?
- is it effective for the learners?
- what are the outcomes for the learners?
- what has been the impact on staff?
- is there the right balance of process, content and product?
- was there any evidence of enjoyment?
- what have the costs really been?
- what have the benefits really been?
- what do employers, colleges or universities think?

Group B identified broad areas for evaluation before generating specific questions, e.g.:

- the quality of classroom/training area experience;
- the organization of the course;
- levels of student motivation and attainment;
- the organizational context for the course.

---

by groups of Certificate of Education students. Which seems the most appropriate to you and why?

In general, Group B's approach is to be recommended simply because it maintains a tight focus on the evaluation work. Even if you have limitless time, money and other resources for evaluation, you still need to be clear about what you are evaluating.

Task 8.12: Deciding what to evaluate in your course

8.12(a)　What is/are the purpose(s) of your evaluation?

8.12(b)　What broad evaluation areas can you identify?

8.12(c)　Why have you decided on these?

Having established the purposes and focal points of the evaluation, what specific issues do you want information about under each of the broad headings and how will you gain this information? The close link between these two is, in reality, a reflection of your educational ideology and the theoretical basis of your course, and this will identify the practical methods of any evaluation. Figure 8.8 presents three theoretical evaluation models to show this. Remember, as with all theoretical models, including those discussed in Chapter 7, you need to use them to help you review and develop your own practice rather than allow them to dictate your approach.

As teachers/trainers, most of us need evaluation data on a range of course issues, both because we want to monitor and improve our work and because others require data for their own purposes. For example, every FE college must collect a wide range of statistical information for the FEFC about levels of recruitment, retention and attainment. This points clearly to you needing to employ a variety of evaluation methods

Figure 8.8 Three models of evaluation

---

1 Scientific evaluation I: classical evaluation

Features:
- views the course as an experiment or treatment to be administered to the students;
- solely interested in measuring course effectiveness defined by the intended outcomes;
- will have test group(s) following the course and control group(s) not following it;
- tests all the students before and after the course to judge course effectiveness and to compare the course with others;
- data and reports very statistical/quantitative.

Figure 8.8 (Cont'd)

This is rather like the late Geoff Hamilton on BBC *Gardeners' World* testing the effectiveness of his organic methods against the use of chemical fertilizers and pesticides. Indeed, classical evaluation is directly descended from these physical science traditions: 'Students, rather like plant crops, are given pre-tests (seedlings being weighed and measured) and then submitted to different experiences. Subsequently, after a period of time, their attainment (growth or yield) is measured to indicate the relative efficiency of the methods (fertilisers etc. used)' (Hamilton 1976: 13).

2 Scientific evaluation II: evaluation via behavioural objectives

Features:
- still views the course as something of an experiment;
- draws on behavioural notions of learning and curriculum design;
- specifies the intended learning outcomes as behavioural objectives;
- records the proportion of students attaining/not attaining the specified behaviours;
- data and reports very statistical/quantitative.

This approach possesses all the advantages and disadvantages of behaviourist perspectives on education and training that were discussed in Chapter 3. For example, can all learning be expressed as behaviours? If not, then this reduces learning to a simplistic shadow of its true nature. However, there is an elegant simplicity to the approach which has seen it become ever more popular in a wide variety of education and training courses.

3 Qualitative evaluation

Features:
- views the course as a human, social activity, not as a scientific experiment;
- interested in a host of content and process issues but especially the course intentions and organization, the experience of the course in practice and the range of outcomes including the unintended;
- also interested in the perspectives of everyone involved, not just the course designer(s);
- uses methods such as observation, interviews and questionnaires as well as assessment and other data;
- reports more language-based than statistical.

This approach draws more on the arts and social sciences so that, rather than aiming for a simple rating of achievement, there is a more complex approach to the measurement of course effectiveness. This means that the aim is to present an holistic picture of the new course in operation which is designed to illuminate the reality of the course for all those involved. Thus, it is hoped, the various strengths and weaknesses might be identified.

(although very few people adopt the classical approach which is more suitable for a formal research project). This variety is certainly acceptable provided, as before, you acknowledge it openly in your course proposal to show you are aware of what you are doing.

> **Task 8.13: In your own words**
>
> 8.13(a) Summarize the main points about these three evaluation models.
>
> 8.13(b) Why, in practice, are a variety of approaches usually adopted?

Now you are in a position to identify what issues you want to evaluate within each of the broad evaluation areas identified in Task 8.12(b) and to specify how information about each could be collected. At this stage, just work through all the issues you would like to evaluate. To help you, Figure 8.9 shows how the same student Group B from Figure 8.7 turned their broad evaluation areas into a series of possible evaluation issues and strategies.

Figure 8.9 Suggested evaluation issues and methods

1 The quality of classroom/training area experience

Specific issues worth evaluating	*Suggested evaluation strategies/ evidence sources (in no order)*

• Purpose
• Pace
• Clarity of teacher talk
• Quality of student activity
• Teaching/learning resources
• Tutor–student and student–student relationships
• Discipline
• Teacher subject knowledge etc.
• Quality of formative and summative assessment strategies
	• Teacher observation
	  – by peer?
	  – by outsider/manager?
	  – by self?
	• Ask the students
	  – verbally?
	  – in writing?
	  – open or closed questions?
	• Teacher qualifications
	• Evidence of record-keeping/ tracking and final success rates

2 The organization of the course

Specific issues worth evaluating	*Suggested evaluation strategies/ evidence sources (in no order)*
• Planning – on the basis of any earlier evaluation? • Resources • Tutorials and support systems	• Evidence of schemes of work and resources available • Course handbook on tutorial and support

Figure 8.9 (Cont'd)

- Staffing
- Monitoring and evaluation procedures

- Evaluation data
- Staffing details
- Evidence of record keeping/ tracking and final success rates
- Ask the students
  - verbally?
  - in writing?
  - open or closed questions?

3 Levels of student motivation and attainment

Specific issues worth evaluating

Suggested evaluation strategies/ evidence sources (in no order)

- Attendance
- Results
- Destinations
- Are students' ideas valued?

- Registers
- Retention rates
- Formal results
- Teacher observation
  - by peer?
  - by outsider/manager?
- Ask the students and note student demeanour, non-verbal behaviour etc.
- Are there any indications of fun, enjoyment, humour etc. demonstrated by staff and students?
- Any earlier evaluation data?

4 The organizational context for the course

Specific issues worth evaluating

Suggested evaluation strategies/ evidence sources (in no order)

- Accommodation
- Resourcing
- Staffing
- Library etc.
- Management and communication

- Visit accommodation, view resources and library
- Ask the students
  - verbally?
  - in writing?
  - open or closed questions?
- Staffing details
- Formal question and answer systems
  - on paper
  - face-to-face

Task 8.14: Identifying specific evaluation issues and methods

Use the suggestions in Figure 8.9 to help your thinking about evaluation.

8.14(a) Select the specific issues you would want to evaluate in your course

8.14(b) Select the evaluation strategies you think would give accurate data.

8.14(c) When would you collect the data? Why is the timing important?

8.14(d) Explain your choices. How practical do you think they are?

8.15(e) Revise your list of issues and strategies in the light of 8.14(d) so that you have a practical as well as an effective evaluation strategy.

Task 8.14(e) raises another major consideration, that of ensuring the evaluation you plan is able to operate in practice. Thus, your original choices in Task 8.14 might well have needed revising. Remember, a small scale, properly thought through and carried out evaluation will be far more useful than a large, impractical and poorly implemented version.

Finally, what will happen to the results of your evaluation? They will need analysing and presenting in a clear format so that the findings can be conveyed to whoever requires them and, more importantly, so that you can identify those areas of the course that need improving and build these into your next course planning session (we should not forget that, in certain circumstances, there may well a good case for not changing things). Whatever the situation, your report must explain the reasons for whatever action or non-action you propose to take.

To summarize, this section has defined course evaluation and has differentiated this from assessment. Evaluation has been presented as a means of judging course effectiveness for a range of interested parties and for a similar range of reasons. Advice has been provided about what to evaluate by suggesting the selection of a small number of key, broad areas as a starting point. Three theoretical models of evaluation have been used to explain the link between what is to be evaluated and how it can be evaluated, followed by an opportunity to make some of these links and to develop a practical and worthwhile evaluation programme. All this is presented as a sequence in Figure 8.10.

Note the final stage. Evaluation is a continuous process if it is to help you keep improving the quality of your course. Moreover, given the moves towards increased accountability in all areas of education and training, as Hopkins (1989) notes, evaluation now often leads to a public discussion and to subsequent action or judgement. There are league tables for almost every aspect of education and training. If we are to engage in evaluation for reasons other than simply our own professionalism, and it seems we must, then any evaluation we carry out must be of

Figure 8.10 Suggested sequence for developing a course evaluation

1 Identify the purpose(s) of the evaluation.
2 Identify the broad areas to be evaluated.
3 Consider the kind(s) of evaluation best suited to your needs.
4 Identify the specific issues to be evaluated and the methods.
5 Ensure the evaluation will be able to operate in practice.
6 Collect the data, analyse, and report to all involved.
7 Explain any proposed changes with reasons.
8 Build changes into next course planning cycle and evaluate.

high quality in order to promote and develop high quality education and training.

 ## *Scrutinizing your course*

KEY ISSUES

Why not allow new and revised courses to operate as soon as they're worked out?

The scrutiny process: what's it all about?

How can a new or revised course be made ready for the scrutiny process?

What does a formal course proposal document contain?

What's involved in presenting a course and in scrutinizing other people's courses?

You might well ask, given all the hard work you have put in already, why you can't just run the course? There are two reasons. First, in line with the notions of increased efficiency and accountability mentioned frequently in this and other chapters, education and training organizations now expect new courses to be developed and presented to set criteria and then examined rigorously and, if necessary, revised, before being allowed to operate. In most colleges and universities, this is called the scrutiny process. National qualifications such as GNVQ and NVQ are offered by awarding bodies and they have a similar process, as do the academic examining boards, for those who wish to develop new or amended versions of such courses.

Second, there is a professional development dimension. Given that we might well have spent time and energy on developing a new course and this might well have been a team effort, there is still a danger that, being so involved and committed to it, we will fail to spot all the flaws in our work. A scrutiny process helps by allowing the organization to take some responsibility for helping us avoid making mistakes. As will be seen later in the section, it also provides us, our colleagues in the organization and in other similar organizations with opportunities to learn about curriculum development by taking part in it. It is the scrutiny process which lies at the heart of this section.

What is the scrutiny process? It is a set of procedures designed to support staff in the development and revision of courses. It ensures that such courses meet the criteria set by the organization and other relevant bodies, are planned to the highest standards, are examined by experts (internal and external to the organization) and are only then allowed to operate.

In most cases, the organization will provide staff with guidelines and some support in the scrutiny process. In this instance, some guidelines are set out in Figure 8.11, while this section and the book as a whole act as support.

Figure 8.11 The scrutiny process

Phase 1: Course development or revision

1.1 The course development team plan what they consider to be an appropriate course following the appropriate framework (NVQ, degree, BTEC rules, police/nurse training regulations etc.).
1.2 The proposed course is organized into a course proposal document and distributed to the others involved in the scrutiny process.

Phase 2: Internal scrutiny

2.1 The course development team makes a formal presentation of their proposed course and document to an internal scrutiny panel composed of the organization's representatives and a number (three?) of staff colleagues acting as internal scrutineers.
2.2 The internal scrutineers use the course document to become familiar with the proposal, listen to the presentation, discuss it and pose searching but not unfriendly questions to the course development team on any issues of concern.
2.3 At the end of this meeting, the internal scrutiny panel must pass one of four judgements on the proposed course:

1 Accept unreservedly in which case the proposal goes forward to Phase 4.
2 Accept subject to minor changes in which case the proposal moves to Phase 3.

Figure 8.11 (Cont'd)

3 Accept subject to major changes in which case the proposal moves to Phase 3.
4 Reject, which means the proposal has no chance of becoming an approved course.

Phase 3: Revisions to original proposal

3.1 Depending on the scale of the changes imposed by the internal scrutiny panel, the course development team works to amend the course proposal in line with the panel's requirements and resubmits a revised course proposal document.
3.2 Once the organization can see that all the necessary changes have been made, the proposal proceeds to the next phase.

Phase 4: External scrutiny

4.1 The scrutiny panel will reconvene but this time with two or three external validators.
4.2 The external validators are specialists in the field but from other organizations. Their role is to carry out an expert and impartial critical scrutiny of the proposed course.
4.3 The course development team makes another formal presentation of their proposed course and document.
4.4 The panel listens to the presentation, discusses it and poses more questions to the course development team on any issues of concern.
4.5 At the end of this meeting, the external scrutiny panel must again pass one of four judgements:

1 Accept unreservedly in which case the proposal goes forward to Phase 5.
2 Accept subject to minor changes in which case the proposal moves to Phase 5 after these changes have been made.
3 Accept subject to major changes in which case the proposal might well need further external scrutiny.
4 Reject, which means that the proposal has lost its chance of becoming an approved course.

Phase 5: Course approved to operate

5.1 The organization will allow the course to be run for up to five years subject to satisfactory levels of recruitment, retention and student success and to satisfactory annual evaluation reports.

What does a course proposal document contain? Figure 8.12 shows the content normally required. In addition, such documents are always presented in as professional a manner as possible. After all, the document represents the quality of your proposed course to those on the scrutiny panels.

Figure 8.12 Contents of a course proposal document

1　A brief rationale for the proposed course explaining why it is such an important development. Add information about student and market needs analysis. Add reasons for sizes of: recruitment targets; minimum and maximum numbers; staff/student ratios.

2　A statement of course aims.

3　An outline of course content expressed as objectives and outcomes.

4　A description of the course organization including: an outline scheme of work; one fully detailed session plan; a typical student's experiences; a typical student's attendance pattern.

5　Details of teaching and learning strategies to be employed.

6　An outline of the assessment framework to be used.

7　An outline of the evaluation framework to be used including sample materials.

8　An indication of any resource implications arising from the new course including accommodation, equipment and staffing (expertise and training as well as number).

9　A costs table including, if possible hourly staffing costs, any other support costs, accommodation and equipment, recurrent costs, overheads etc. These are usually available from organizations' administrators.

10　An indication of revenue from the course showing sources and levels both short and (estimated) longer term together with some comment as to how certain and long-lasting the revenue might be.

Task 8.15: The scrutiny process: what's it all about?

8.15(a)　Why shouldn't we just put our new courses straight into operation?

8.15(b)　What are the purposes of a scrutiny process?

8.15(c)　How does it work and what is the role of the course proposal document?

This all looks like a pretty large piece of work, and so it is. This is a full course proposal and getting a new or revised course off the ground is a serious business. So, how can you make what you already have produced in terms of your new or revised course into a formal course proposal ready to go forward to the scrutiny process? For quick reference, Table 8.2 links each task from Chapters 7 and 8 with sections in the course proposal document.

Table 8.2 Tasks linked to creating a course proposal document

Proposal document content	Section	Task	Course development activity
1, 2, 3, 4, 5, 6, 7	7.5	7.14	Sharpen thinking on curriculum, ideology, curriculum models
1, 2, 3	8.2	8.1	Identify your curriculum development or revision task
1, 2, 3	8.2	8.2	Decide on the kind of course it will be
8, 9, 10	8.2	8.3	Identify the organization's criteria for costs, numbers, etc.
2	8.2	8.4	Conduct a needs analysis
1, 2, 3	8.2	8.5	Decide on the broad purposes for the course
2, 3	8.2	8.6	Specify the course aims and objectives
4, 5, 6	8.2	8.7, 8.8, 8.9	Specify content, sequence, learning/assessment experiences
7	8.3	8.10, 8.11, 8.12, 8.13, 8.14	Establish a set of evaluation procedures

Task 8.16: Writing most of your course proposal document

8.16(a) Using Table 8.2 collect all your responses to earlier tasks together.

8.16(b) Write them up in full and arrange them under the ten headings of a course proposal document, as outlined in Figure 8.12.

You should find that the only areas requiring further work are 8, 9 and 10 on resources, costs and revenue. Once again, don't worry. Even if you hate working with figures Task 8.17 will show you how to tackle this area.

Task 8.17: Writing the rest of your course proposal document

Your own organization will have ready-made lists of costs for most kinds of course and will usually help refine these for your particular course. Ask for their standard costings and for additional advice if needed.

If you are hoping to run a self-financing course, hotels, conference centres and other venues all provide cost schedules on request. Just ask for them.

Revenue is more a matter of estimation. Work out what income you expect the course to generate and consider how certain you are of your figures and for how long you expect revenue to be earned. Write this up including the basis for your estimates. Ask your organization for help if you need it – they should be used to assisting their staff with this kind of issue.

8.17(a) Write up your work on these areas and add to your course proposal document.

8.17(b) Check through your document to ensure that every heading is complete and that the spelling, layout and general feel of the document is as professional (not flashy) as possible.

Finally, what is involved in being a presenter and a scrutineer at one of these scrutiny panel meetings? In order to gain for yourself the maximum quantity and quality of professional benefit from this chapter, you are strongly advised to work with at least one other person to reproduce a scrutiny process for yourself. If you are a member of a group, all the better. Several of you can work together to develop a proposal, perhaps starting with one person's idea or a real course development task someone has been given. Others can act as scrutineers of that group's proposal. Then you can reverse the roles.

In essence, what is being asked of you is to work from two perspectives: that of the curriculum developer and that of the scrutiny panel member. Things can often look different from someone else's perspective and you will learn a great deal by having your own course development scrutinized by someone else and by scrutinizing someone else's course proposal yourself. It will also be invaluable preparation for working on similar tasks in your teaching and training work. Indeed, a fair proportion of Certificate of Education course proposals become real courses and go into operation very smoothly because of their careful planning and preparation. To help you to prepare for a scrutiny panel meeting, Figures 8.13 and 8.14 provide guidance on how to be a member of a scrutiny panel and how to be a course presenter.

In order for scrutiny panel members to operate as effectively as possible, a sample checklist and form is provided in Figure 8.15. This would normally be printed over two sides of an A4 sheet and completed copies would be given to the presenters as well as to the organization's representatives.

Task 8.18: Preparing for a scrutiny panel

If you are able to attend a scrutiny panel meeting, either as a presenter or as a scrutineer, use Figures 8.13, 8.14 and 8.15 to help you prepare for the event.

Figure 8.13 Being a scrutiny panel member

The role of a scrutiny panel member is:

- to complete a comprehensive evaluation of the proposal focusing on the use of curriculum ideology and design model(s) as well as evaluating the proposal as set out in Figure 8.12;
- to help the course development team to make progress and suggest action points as needed (unless the proposal is a non-starter, in which case the organization should have stopped it earlier);
- harder than it might seem!

We must therefore be critical where necessary, award praise where appropriate and, above all, be positive. We are there to help another set of professionals with their work, not to turn it into our work!

Tasks of a scrutiny panel member

- Before the scrutiny panel meeting to read the course proposal document thoroughly and draw up a checklist of questions and comments.
- During the scrutiny panel meeting to listen to the presentation and delete or add questions and comments to the checklist.
- Immediately following the presentation to ask questions of clarification.
- During the post-presentation discussion to ask questions, discuss and provide feedback in a critical and/or positive manner as appropriate, perhaps by always having a positive suggestion to make following any criticism. If changes are needed, the job is to help them be made, not simply point out the problem.

Figure 8.14 Being a course presenter at a scrutiny panel

The role of a course presenter is:

- to provide as professional a proposal document as possible well in advance of the meeting;
- to provide evidence of depth of information and thinking through the presentation;
- harder than it might seem!

We must, therefore, plan and prepare for the presentation very carefully. We are there to help other professionals to gain an accurate picture of our proposals, not to 'sock it to 'em'!

Tasks of a course presenter

- Before the scrutiny panel meeting to supply sufficient copies of a high-quality course proposal document.
- To plan and deliver a professional presentation. There will usually be at least 20 minutes for your presentation and plenty of time for discussion and for the scrutineers' questions afterwards.

Figure 8.14 (Cont'd)

- To ensure that the style of the presentation reflects the course: give a sample of how students will experience it and use any techniques you feel are appropriate. Above all make it interesting (and fun!).
- During the scrutiny panel meeting to listen as well as talk, and not be too defensive.
- Immediately following the presentation to answer questions of clarification.
- During the post-presentation discussion to answer questions, discuss and respond to feedback as appropriate, avoiding defensiveness and always having a positive approach to the meeting. If need be, ask for positive action points to follow any criticism. Remember, if changes are needed, the job of the scrutiny panel is to help to develop the course.

Figure 8.15 Suggestions for a scrutiny panel evaluation form

Presenting team:

Course title and details:

Scrutiny panel criteria:
Use the following checklist to make brief notes here as needed.

1 Is there a brief rationale for the proposed course? Does it include:
- a student and market needs analysis?
- recruitment targets?
- minimum and maximum numbers?
- staff/student ratios?

2 Is there a statement of course aims and objectives? Are these appropriate to the needs of the client group? Do they specify the kinds of intended learning outcomes?

3 Is there an outline of course content which is linked to the intended aims/objectives/outcomes?

4 Is there a description of the course organization, an outline scheme of work and a session plan, outlines of staff/student ratios, and a typical student's experiences and attendance pattern?

5 Are there details of teaching and learning strategies/materials to be employed which seem to match the intended aims/objectives/outcomes?

6 Is the assessment framework to be used appropriate to the intended aims etc.?

7 Is the evaluation framework to be used appropriate to the intended aims etc.?

8 Is there evidence that the following have been considered?
- resource implications;
- costs;
- revenue.

Figure 8.15 (Cont'd)

General comments and any recommended revisions/additions:

Overall recommendation (delete as appropriate):

- Accept now
- Accept with minor/major revisions as specified above
- Reject

Name of scrutineer:

Date:

To summarize, this section has examined the process through which most organizations now support and approve the development and revision of new courses. The scrutiny process has been explained and a framework provided for the new course to be presented as a single document. Furthermore, explicit links have been made between this final document and the tasks spread through this chapter so that readers are able to see how their work can contribute to a full course proposal.

Finally, the section has advised all readers to take part in the scrutiny process or something similar because of the tremendous amount of professional learning that will emerge from such an experience. To this end, guidance and advice have been provided covering both the roles of course presenter and scrutineer.

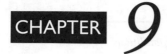

CHAPTER *9*

DEVELOPMENTS IN POST-COMPULSORY EDUCATION

9.1 *What is Chapter 9 about?*

Teachers and trainers in PCE may teach specialist subjects but they may also see themselves as educators or even educationalists and seek to become knowledgeable about the subject of education. This view is rather unpopular and may even seem indulgent. Teaching is seen more and more as a practical activity in which experience is valued over theoretical knowledge. Competence-based teacher training programmes and the governmental obsession with school discipline means that the subject-based teacher education programmes of the 1970s no longer exist. As we saw in Chapter 1, the new educational thought of that time resulted in ideas, theories and clear distinctions that are now thought to constitute arid rationalism. Chapter 1 examined the problematic nature of teaching in the post-compulsory sector, and focused particularly on developing post-compulsory teachers' understanding of the various educational philosophies that influence their professional practice. These views were related to well-known theories of learning. This chapter complements Chapter 1 in a broader way. It will provide the post-compulsory teacher with the essential background to begin to examine the contemporary historical development of PCE.

Teachers sometimes like to think that their subject and/or vocation, whatever they like to call it, stands on its own without regard to outside influences or broader trends in society. Nothing could be further from the truth. Any consideration of the nature of education or its translation into the sphere of policy is the result of a much more complex set of relations in society. This does not have to be a one-way street from broader social trends to education policy nor is it a process devoid of contradiction. Serious thinking and passionately held beliefs about education will themselves have an impact on the way that society thinks about itself and there will often be a gap between intention and outcome. Nevertheless the way education is viewed will say a great deal about the society as a whole.

It is in the very nature of education that it will be emblematic of how society both would like itself to be and how it hopes and aspires to get there. In general then, it should be no surprise that discussion about education often preoccupies discussion about issues as apparently wide-ranging as economic performance and moral rectitude. The significance of the discussion for us is not at this level of generality but in the specific combination of argument, interest, problems and solutions that we find in the development of PCE in the post-war period in Britain.

We would argue that any professional practitioner must have such knowledge if they are to be purposeful and active participants in their own professional development and the development of their profession. Otherwise those that do have that knowledge will merely direct them without them having the benefit of the informed discussion and debate that is essential to the practice of education. However, we recognize that many post-compulsory teachers will not have the background in educational history, social policy or related studies to give them a sufficient knowledge base to make a conscious contribution to debate. This chapter has been designed around a series of activities that present opposing views and interpretations which, we believe, uncover the issues at the heart of contemporary debates and will provide clear critical guidelines for further discussion.

Section 9.2 introduces the chronology of PCE in England and Wales presented in Section 9.3 which gives the reader a broad survey of major developments. Even readers familiar with PCE and its history might like to skim-read this chronology before reading later sections. Section 9.4 introduces a short comparative chronology looking at developments in PCE in the USA as presented in Section 9.5.

9.2 *The purpose of the chronology*

What follows is an overview of major government reports, education acts, and important developments relating to PCE which provide the essential historical background to the analysis of the issues discussed in previous chapters. Emphasis is given to developments in the post-Second World War period, although major developments relating to education since the industrial revolution are also summarized. The purpose is to provide the reader with basic factual information in a concise and accessible form. Authorial commentary and discussion has been largely omitted but the selection has a deliberate focus on developments in FE and youth training. We do not hide the fact that it is a central part of our argument that developments in this latter area are now influencing education at all levels. Developments in the general educational sphere, in AE, HE and in special education are also listed if these are essential to the identification of educational trends.

Reading the chronology

A chronology is simply a list of events in date order. We are using the term to describe a carefully selected list to give the reader an overview of key events, reports, acts and writings in the history of PCE. The best way to approach the chronology is to skim-read the dates and headings in bold. Then go back through the whole document reading complete sections or entries of interest. The tasks are in the form of questions to guide your thinking about historical periods.

Reflecting on the chronology

To make sense of the chronology we suggest two methods of reflection. The first is to think in terms of what different generations of young people might have expected or experienced of post-compulsory education or training in any specific historical period. The second approach is to step back from the details of the particular discussion or development in PCE and attempt to locate young people's expectations in the wider context of social policy and political and economic events.

Boxes within the text contain relevant political and economic facts to remind the reader of the historical context of the events listed. The interaction between these three activities (getting familiar with particular events, imagining the expectations of generations of young people and locating these in a wider social context) are essential to understanding.

9.3   *A chronology of post-compulsory education*

1563: Statute of Artificers. This statute established the seven-year apprenticeship as the basic form of training in England. A further act, the Poor Law of 1601, allowed for the forcible apprenticeship of pauper children. Craft apprenticeship was the form of technical training up to the time of the industrial revolution. Arguably, it remained the dominant form of work-related training up to the 1960s when the Industrial Training Act (1964) was passed.

1823: Mechanics' institutes established. Mechanics' institutes were set up in Chester in 1810, Perth in 1814, Edinburgh in 1821 (actually a 'school of arts') and most famously in Glasgow in 1823. George Birkbeck taught at what was to become the Glasgow Mechanics Institute but left to practise as a physician in London. He helped establish a similar institute there in 1823 which was to become Birkbeck College. The movement grew and had its own publication *The Mechanic's Magazine*. By 1826 there were 110 institutes and by 1850 some 600,000 people were attending classes in one of 610 institutes.

1846: pupil–teacher system introduced. Bright pupils were apprenticed at 13 years of age to head teachers for a period of five years.

1856: Royal Society of Arts (RSA) founds first national examining board.

1856: Education Department formed. Robert Lowe became vice-president in 1859 and introduced the system of 'payment by results' which lasted until 1900. Grants were given on the basis of school attendance, which was revealed to be low by the Newcastle Commission Report of 1861, and on the results of an examination in the 'three Rs'.

1864: Clarendon Commission Report. The commission suggested that the classical curriculum of the public schools be supplemented by instruction in subjects such as mathematics and science.

1868: Taunton Commission Report. The commission emphasized the importance of natural science as a subject because it was seen as of value in 'occupations'. The commissioners outlined various 'grades' of education ending respectively at 14 (Grade 3), 16 (Grade 2), and 18 (Grade 1), meeting the needs of the various social classes.

1870: Elementary Education Act (Forster Act). The Great Education Act introduced a national system of elementary education for children up to 13 years of age replacing the previous system based on 'voluntary schools'. School boards became responsible for the running of the new 'Board Schools' and pupil attendance was at their discretion. Fees were charged. The Education Act of 1880 had to be passed to attempt to make elementary education compulsory by requiring school boards to enact by-laws to this effect. Employment of children under 10 was made illegal under the Factory and Workshops Act of 1878. Introducing the act Forster told the Commons: 'Upon the speedy provision of elementary education depends our industrial prosperity' (Maclure 1965: 104).

Task 9.1

Consider what sort of education a young person would receive at this time. Why should an educational debate about the suitability of an education based upon the classics or one extended to include more relevant subjects such as mathematics or science arise in the 1860s? Why should there be only an 'elementary' education act passed at this time and why one that provided an education which was neither universal nor free?

Education in context: 1868–1922

Prime ministers: 1868 Disraeli (Conservative); 1868–74 Gladstone (Liberal); 1874–80 Disraeli II (Conservative); 1880–5 Gladstone (Liberal); 1885–6 Gascoyne-Cecil, 3rd Marquis of Salisbury (Conservative); 1886 Gladstone (Liberal); 1886–92 Gascoyne-Cecil, 3rd Marquis of Salisbury (Conservative); 1892–4 Gladstone (Liberal); 1894–5 5th Earl of Rosebery (Liberal); 1895–1902 Gascoyne-Cecil, 3rd Marquis of Salisbury (Conservative); 1902–5 Balfour (Conservative); 1905–8 Campbell Bannerman (Liberal); 1908–16 Asquith (Liberal/coalition); 1916–22 Lloyd George (Liberal/coalition).

Presidents of the board of education: from January 1900, Duke of Devonshire; from August 1902, Marquis of Londonderry; from December 1905, A. Birrell; from January 1907, R. McKenna; from April 1908, W. Runciman; from October 1911, J. Pease; from May 1915, A. Henderson; from August 1916, Marquis of Crewe; from December 1916, H. Fisher.

Key political and economic events: 1851 Great Exhibition; 1867 Paris Exhibition, Reform Act; 1868 Trades Union Congress formed; 1870–1 Franco-PrussianWar; 1873 'Great Depression'; 1883 Depression, Fabian Society formed; 1887 Jubilee; 1889 first skyscraper in Chicago; 1897 Diamond Jubilee; 1898 Spanish American War, match girls strike; 1889 London dock strike; 1899–1902 Second Boer War; 1903 Ford Motor Company founded; 1914–18 First World War; 1917 Russian Revolution.

1879: the City & Guilds of London Institute (CGLI) founded in 1878 is given the responsibility for technical examining from the RSA.

1880: The famous Regent Street Polytechnic founded. One of many in different parts of Britain which developed out of the Mechanics' Institutes.

1882–4: Samuelson Committee. This committee made recommendations about the need for scientific and technical instruction of the sort that was already available to workers in America and many European countries.

1889: Technical Instruction Act. This enabled the new counties and county councils to provide technical education. A transfer of tax reserves popularly known as 'whisky money' was used mostly to provide science education.

1890: day training colleges for teachers are introduced.

1902: Education Act (Balfour Act). When introducing his bill in the house Balfour stressed the need for a sound general education. There was already a single supervisory body for education in existence at a national level. This was the Board of Education that had been formed by an act of 1899. Actual provision of education at a local level became the responsibility of local education authorities (LEAs) which took over the powers of the school boards. They were required to form education committees. Pupils could now stay on in an elementary school up to 16 years of age and beyond. LEAs had powers to train teachers.

1903: the Association for the Higher Education of Working Men founded. It became the Workers' Educational Association (WEA) in 1905. By 1968 the WEA was catering for 150,000 students and had 85 full-time staff (WEA evidence to the Russell Report 1973).

1906: Haldane Committee Report on technical education. The report called for the establishment of a group of colleges of science and technology where the highest specialized instruction could be given. The result was the founding of Imperial College in 1907.

1907: Ruskin Hall (1899) became Ruskin College, Oxford. Its founding document states that the college is 'designed to equip the workers for the struggle against capitalism and capitalist ideology'.

Education in context: 1922–45

Prime ministers: 1922–3 Bonar Law (Conservative); 1923–4 Baldwin (Conservative); 1924 MacDonald (Labour); 1924–9 Baldwin (Conservative); 1929–35 MacDonald (Labour/coalition); 1935–7 Baldwin (National); 1937–40 Chamberlain (National); 1940–5 Churchill (coalition).

Presidents of the board of education: from October 1922, E. Wood; from January 1924, C. Trevelyan; from November 1924, Lord Percy; from June 1929, Sir C. Trevelyan; from March 1931, H. Lees Smith; from August 1931, Sir D. Maclean; from June 1932, Lord Irwin (Viscount Halifax); from June 1935, O. Stanley; from May 1937, Earl Stanhope; from October 1938, Earl De La Warr; from April 1940, H. Ramsbotham; from July 1941, R. Butler.

Ministers of education: from August 1944, R. Butler; from May 1945, R. Law.

Key political and economic events: 1924 first Labour government; 1926 General Strike; 1929 Wall Street crash, Depression; 1931 Empire State Building completed; 1933 Hitler becomes chancellor of Germany; 1936–9 Spanish Civil War; 1939–45 Second World War.

1917: School Certificate introduced.

1918: Education Act (Fisher Act). The school leaving age was raised to 14 with most pupils staying in all-age elementary schools. Fees were abolished. Central government would meet not less than half the costs of educational provision. Young workers should have a right to day release. Many other things 'allowed' but not compelled by the act fell when funding was cut by one-third in 1922 ('Geddes axe'). Introducing his Education Bill on 10 August 1917, H.A.L. Fisher, the architect of the 1918 act, argued that 'education is one of the good things of life' and that the 'principles upon which well-to-do parents proceed in the education of their families are valid; also *mutatis mutandis* for the families of the poor' (Maclure 1965: 175).

1922: R.H. Tawney's *Secondary Education for All* **published.**

1926: Evening Institutes established. The precursors of AE institutes and colleges, these, along with the technical schools provided most of the technical education available in the inter-war period.

1926: Hadow Report *The Education of the Adolescent.* The Hadow Committee recommended a broad and balanced secondary school curriculum which prepared students for diverse occupational groups. It called for the establishment of 'modern' or 'central' schools and 'grammar' schools for pupils with different gifts. Hadow subsequently headed committees that reported on the primary school (1931) and the nursery and infant school (1933).

1938: Spens Report. The *Report of the Consultative Committee on Secondary Education* was strongly supportive of the idea of 'technical high schools' which would not be narrowly vocational but equal in status to grammar schools. The basis for the post-war tripartite system was now set. Spens also suggested changes to the curriculum, the School Certificate and the matriculation system.

1939–45: day release expands from 42,000 to 150,000 during the Second World War.

1940: the Department of Education publishes its 'Green Book' *Education after the War.*

1942: Beveridge Report. This set out plans for a comprehensive system of social security 'from the cradle to the grave'.

1943: White Paper *Educational Reconstruction.* This set out a vision of an educational system after the war which would provide for diversity while ensuring equality of educational opportunity.

1943: Norwood Report. In a report about examinations appeared proposals for a system of selection through intelligence testing for entry into a tripartite secondary education system made up of modern, technical and grammar secondary schools.

1944: McNair Report. McNair proposed three-year training courses for teachers. The report suggested that training for technical teachers should commence after rather than before they started to practise as teachers.

Task 9.2

This task should be in written form, either as short essays or as a group activity using flip charts. Discuss the period from 1870–1945 with your fellow students. What would school leavers expect to receive in terms of PCE during this period? Construct brief educational biographies of people who would have been in their late teens in, for example, 1880, 1910 and 1930. Having done this identify the key characteristics of British education over the period from 1870 to 1913 and between the two World Wars (1918–1939). Comment on how you think this reflects the position of Britain in the world and its economic situation during the two periods. You might like to consider why 1870 is considered to be an economic turning point for Britain.

Education in context: 1945–51

Prime minister: 1945–51 Clement Atlee (Labour).

Ministers of education: from August 1945, Ellen Wilkinson; from February 1947, George Tomlinson.

Key political and economic events: 1945 United Nations established; 1947 European reconstruction (Marshall Plan); 1950–3 Korean War; 1950 Britain is the economic leader in Europe; 1951 Festival of Britain.

1944: Education Act (Butler Act). This made provision of primary, secondary and FE a duty. A clause allowed for the possibility of compulsory (part-time) further education for all young people up to the age of 18. It was, however, only to become compulsory on a day to be decided. The school leaving age was to be raised to 15.

1945: Percy Report. Entitled *Higher Technological Education*, the report looked at how universities were responding to the needs of industry.

Education in context: 1951–64

Prime ministers: 1951–5 Winston Churchill (Conservative); 1955–7 Sir Anthony Eden (Conservative); 1957–63 Harold Macmillan (Conservative); 1963–4 Sir Alec Douglas-Home (Conservative).

Ministers of education: from November 1951, Florence Horsburgh; from October 1954, Sir David Eccles; from January 1957, Viscount Hailsham; from September 1957, Geoffrey Lloyd; from October 1959, Sir David Eccles; from July 1962, Sir Edward Boyle. The Ministry of Education became the Department of Education and Science (DES) in April 1964 with Quintin Hogg as secretary of state for education and science.

Key political and economic events: the post-war economic boom; the cold war; anti-colonial struggles in the Third World; 1952 Mau Mau rebellion in Kenya; 1953 Organization of African Unity formed; 1956 Hungarian Revolution; 1956 Suez crisis, Vietnam War begins; 1957 Treaty of Rome, European Economic Community (EEC) formed; 1961 Berlin Wall; 1962 Cuban missile crisis.

1945: Emergency Training Scheme introduced. The aim of this was to increase the supply of teachers. After much criticism, it ended in 1951.

1951: General Certificate of Education (GCE) introduced. The GCE replaced the much criticized School Certificate.

1956: White Paper *Technical Education.*

1957: Willis Jackson Report *The Training of Technical Teachers.*

1959: Crowther Report *15–18.* The report looked at the different educational needs of a technological age. It noted that over 40 per cent of LEAs had no technical schools. For those who got 'incurably tired of school' the report argued for a 'fresh start in a technical college or some other quasi-adult institution' (HMSO 1959: 412). Specialization in-depth was necessary in the sixth form but not on the basis of vocational usefulness. Crowther recommended that the school leaving age be raised to 16. By 1980 it was hoped that half of 16–18-year-olds should be in full-time FE.

1960: the Further Education Staff College founded at Coombe Lodge, Blagdon, near Bristol.

1963: 'University of the Air' called for in a speech by Harold Wilson. Wilson told his biographer that this was what he wanted to be remembered for 'above almost anything else in his career' (Timmins 1996: 300).

1963: Robbins Report *Higher Education.* 'Throughout our report we have assumed as an axiom that courses of higher education should be available for all who are qualified by ability and attainment to pursue them and who wish to do so'(Maclure 1965: 297). Robbins set out a vision of how HE could expand. He suggested an increase from 8 per cent of the school leaving population to 17 per cent by 1980. The report resulted in the setting up of the Council for National Academic Awards (CNAA) and made the training of teachers a responsibility of HE. Teacher training colleges were renamed Colleges of Education. Colleges of advanced technology (CATs) became university institutions.

Task 9.3

The 1960s was a decade of influential reports. Two others of note are the Newsom Report *Half Our Future* (1963) which suggested that schools should offer a more modern education relevant to the experiences of pupils of below average ability, and the Plowden Report *Children and their Primary Schools* (1967) which put the case for child-centred education. A reaction came at the end of the decade with the publication of the *Black Papers* on education in 1969 and 1975 which argued for a return to formal methods of teaching, grammar schooling and hard-working academic students at university level. Consider what PCE would be available to young people in the latter half of the decade. What is special about the 1960s that made it a decade of political and educational consensus?

Education in context: 1964–70

Prime minister: 1964–70 Harold Wilson (Labour).

Secretaries of state for education and science: from October 1964, Michael Stewart; from January 1965, Anthony Crosland; from August 1967, Patrick Gordon Walker; from April 1968, Edward Short.

Key political and economic events: post-war political consensus: economic and industrial 'modernization' becomes a theme; The Beatles; Vietnam War; 1964 (USA) Civil Rights Bill; 1968 student protests, Organization of Arab petroleum Exporting Countries (OAPEC) formed; 1969 first man on the moon.

1964: the Certificate of Secondary Education (CSE) introduced. Council for National Academic Awards (CNAA) established.

1964: Industrial Training Boards (ITBs). These boards were established by the minister of labour as a consequence of the Industrial Training Act of the same year. The ITBs were meant to improve the quality of training and thus tackle the problem of real craft skill shortages. Administered by employers and trade union representatives the ITBs covered most of the large industrial employment sectors. Within seven years there were '27 ITBs covering employers with some 15 million workers' (Finn 1987: 56).

1969: Open University founded.

Education in context: 1970–4

Prime minister: 1970–4 Edward Heath (Conservative).

Secretary of state for education and science: from June 1970, Margaret Thatcher.

Key political and economic events: 1971 collapse of the Bretton Woods agreement, President Nixon formally ended convertibility of gold 'on demand' with the dollar; 1973 miners' strike, oil crisis, three-day week, Britain joins the EEC; 1974–5 world economic recession.

1970: Education (Handicapped Children) Act. A hundred years after the great Elementary Education Act, children categorized as 'severely subnormal' and considered 'ineducable' were brought out of junior training schools and into the education system.

1970: first tertiary college founded in Devon. The development of tertiary colleges had been argued for by several influential figures including Tessa Blackstone.

1971: Open University enrols its first students.

1972: James Report. This report suggested three stages of teacher training. A two-year Diploma in Higher Education followed by a year of professional studies based in school. This would lead to the award of the BA (Ed.).

1972: school leaving age raised to 16 from September.

1972: *Training for the Future* (DE). This White Paper highlighted failures in the 1964 Industrial Training Act and called for the phasing out of the training levy and for a new role for ITBs. It set up the Training Opportunities Scheme (TOPS).

1973: Technician Education Council (TEC) and Business Education Council (BEC) set up. This was as a result of the 1969 Haslegrave Report to plan, coordinate and administer technical courses and examinations.

1973: Russell Report *Adult Education: A Plan for Development.* As the title suggests Russell argued for an expansion of non-vocational AE, particularly because of the unmet needs of 'school-leavers and young adults, older adults, the handicapped and "the disadvantaged"'. Russell set the tone for much of the subsequent debate about AE.

1973: Manpower Services Commission (MSC). The MSC was set up under the Employment and Training Act (1973) to supervise employment and with sufficient powers to plan training at national level. The MSC assumed its responsibilities on 1 January 1974.

1973: Haycocks Report (Haycocks I) on the training of full-time FE teachers. The report made major recommendations for improved training. The government in Circular 11/77 welcomed the proposals and supported the in-service training of 3 per cent of staff at any one time. The report was followed in March 1978 by Haycocks II on AE and part-time teachers and in August 1978 by Haycocks III on the training of FE teachers for 'education management'.

Education in context: 1974–9

Prime ministers: 1974–6 Harold Wilson (Labour); 1976–9 James Callaghan (Labour).

Secretaries of state for education and science: from March 1994 , Reg Prentice; from June 1975, Fred Mulley; from September 1976, Shirley Williams.

Key political and economic events: sterling crisis, IMF intervention, stagflation (inflation and high unemployment); 1975 Vietnam War ends, civil war in the Lebanon; 1978 Egypt and Israel sign the Camp David Treaty; 1979 Islamic Republic established in Iran, 'winter of discontent' in Britain.

1976: the Great Debate. Prime Minister James Callaghan delivers a speech *'Towards a national debate'* on 18 October 1976 at Ruskin College, Oxford. This speech has been described as 'a beacon in the history of post-war education. It brought education into the full light of public debate, giving education a position of prominence on public agendas where it has remained ever since' (Williams 1992: 1–2).

One question that Callaghan was addressing had been set for him by Fred Mulley (secretary of state for education and science from June 1975): what was available for the 16–19-year-olds? One concern was the over specialization at A level. In the speech the goal of education was said to be 'to equip children to the best of their ability for a lively constructive place in society and also to fit them to do a job of work'. Emphasis must be given to 'not one or the other, but both'. One passage is worth quoting as it could have been a statement made by any education minister, secretary of state for education, prime minister or member of the opposition since then:

> Let me repeat some of the fields that need study because they cause concern. There are the methods and aims of informal instruction: the strong case for the so-called 'core curriculum' of basic knowledge; next, what is the proper way of monitoring the use of resources in order to maintain a proper national standard of performance; then there is the role of the Inspectorate in relation to national standards; and there is the need to improve relations between industry and education.
>
> (Maclure 1988: 169)

The Great Debate itself centred around eight days of debate organized at a regional level and led by the DES. A White Paper *Education for Schools* published in 1977 summarized the debate.

Task 9.4

Claims about the importance of historical figures and their speeches are often made. To understand why Callaghan's speech is held to be exceptional the economic context must be examined. Some thinkers argue that the reasons for the revival of vocationalism since the 1970s are 'primarily economic' (Skilbeck *et al.* 1994: 1). Try to identify these economic factors. Begin by asking what educational opportunities would young people expect in the middle and late 1970s.

1977: The Holland Report *Young People and Work* (MSC). The aim of the Holland Report was 'building a better workforce more adapted to the needs of the eighties'. It proposed work experience and work preparation courses for unemployed young people. They would be paid a weekly allowance. It proposed the setting up of the Youth Opportunities Programme (YOP) which began in 1978.

1977: The FEU set up as a curriculum development and dissemination body for FE. It was originally called the Further Education Curriculum Review and Development Unit. Although it was a quasi-autonomous body, the FEU was funded by the DES.

1978: The Warnock Report *Special Educational Needs.* Warnock abolished the various categories of handicap then in use and suggested a wider more individualized concept of special needs which was to be enshrined in the 1981 Education Act.

Education in context: 1979–90

Prime minister: 1979–90 Margaret Thatcher (Conservative).

Secretaries of state for education and science: from May 1979, Mark Carlisle; from September 1981, Sir Keith Joseph; from May 1986, Kenneth Baker; from July 1989, John MacGregor.

Key political and economic events: monetarism (controlling inflation by controlling the money supply), Thatcherism (the manifestation of this in the Thatcher government), privatization (denationalization of industry and government); 1982 Falklands War; 1984 miners' strike; 1987 stock market crash, 'There is no such thing as society' (Margaret Thatcher); 1989 fall of Berlin Wall, collapse of Communist regimes in Eastern Europe.

1979: *A Basis for Choice* (FEU). This report emphasized the need for a 'common core' curriculum which emphasized transferable skills and flexibility through participating in 'learning experiences' rather than narrow skills-based teaching.

1981: *A New Training Initiative* (NTI). The MSC produced two documents *A New Training Initiative: A Consultative Document* in May 1981 and later in December *A New Training Initiative: An Agenda for Action.* These documents set the training agenda for the decade. Skills training for young people and adults was covered.

1982: *17+ A New Qualification* (DES). This document set out the basis for the introduction of the CPVE for students who had not yet chosen their vocation.

1983: TVEI starts. Announced by Mrs Thatcher in November 1982 it was to be the largest curriculum intervention ever by a government. The scheme was under the control of the MSC. It was a broad and experimental scheme aimed at preparing 14–18-year-olds for the world of work and developing personal qualities such as enterprise and 'problem solving' skills.

1983: YTS. YTS replaced YOP. In 1988 there were over half a million contracted YTS places and an average of 370,00 students in training.

1983: Business and Technology Education Council (BTEC) formed through the merger of BEC and TEC.

1984: White Paper *Training for Jobs*. This made clear the government's intention to make the MSC the 'national training authority'. A report: *Competence and Competition* by the National Economic Development Office (NEDO)/MSC saw the competitive success of Japan, Germany and the USA was seen as being related to their investment in education.

1985: Further Education Act. Allowed colleges to engage in commercial activities related to areas of expertise and generate more funding. Governors were made responsible for the college budgets.

1985: CPVE introduced. It was never successful even with less able pupils and take-up was poor.

1986: NCVQ established on 1 October. Only 40 per cent of the workforce held relevant qualifications. Despite the 'tremendous expansion in training', this was still a much lower proportion than in other countries. NCVQ's primary task was 'to reform and rationalise the provision of vocational qualifications through the creation of the National Vocational Qualification Framework' (NCVQ 1988: 1). The NCVQ introduced through the awarding bodies (RSA, CGLI etc.) competence-based NVQs that were based in the workplace and not just work-related.

1987: Enterprise in Higher Education Initiative (EHEI). Seen as the HE equivalent of TVEI this initiative had a budget of £100 million. The aim was to see every person in HE developing 'competencies and aptitudes relevant to enterprise'.

1988: the General Certificate of Secondary Education (GCSE) replaces the GCE and CSE.

1988: Education Reform Act (ERA). This Act, which followed from Kenneth Baker's so-called Great Education Reform Bill sought to revitalize the 'producer dominated' education system (Maclure 1988: iv). ERA brought in the National Curriculum for schools with core subjects (English, mathematics, science and religious education) to be learned by all. Several cross-curriculum themes were also identified: environmental education; education for citizenship; careers education and guidance; health education; and economic and industrial understanding. It also had a strong emphasis on moral renewal seeking to promote 'the spiritual, moral, cultural, mental and physical development of pupils at the school and of society' (Maclure 1988: 1). The act delegated financial responsibilities from local authorities to schools. It took polytechnics out of local authority control and replaced the National Advisory Body for Public Sector Higher Education with the Polytechnics and Colleges Funding Council. It required that half of the membership of the governing bodies of FE colleges represented employment interests.

1988: The MSC absorbed into the Department of Employment (DoE), becoming the Training Commission for a short time and then the Training Agency.

1989: The Confederation of British Industry (CBI) publishes *Towards a Skills Revolution.* This advocated common learning outcomes for all students over 16. This document set out the employers' agenda for lifelong learning.

1989: Kenneth Baker calls for a doubling of the numbers of students entering HE in a speech at Lancaster University. Numbers should increase to 30 per cent. This was achieved by the mid-1990s.

1989: YTS replaced by Youth Training (YT).

Task 9.5

Discussions of the YTS and the role of the MSC dominated educational thought during the 1980s. Why was this? Again, it might be useful to construct an educational biography of a young person brought up in the time of the first Thatcher government.

Education in context: 1990–7

Prime ministers: 1990–7 John Major (Conservative); 1997– Tony Blair (Labour).

Secretary of state for education and science: from November 1990, Kenneth Clarke.

Secretaries of state for education: from April 1992, John Patten; from July 1994, Gillian Shepherd.

Secretaries of state for education and employment: from July 1995, Gillian Shepherd; from May 1997 David Blunkett. Baroness Tessa Blackstone was given responsibility for education and employment in the House of Lords. Professor Michael Barber of the University of London Institute of Education made director of a newly-formed Standards and Performance Unit, a hit squad for failing schools and teachers.

Key political and economic events: economic recession, Citizen's Charters, social authoritarianism; 1991 the Gulf War, civil war in Yugoslavia; 1992 United Nations (UN) intervention in Somalia and Bosnia.

1990: Core Skills 16–19 published by National Curriculum Council (NCC) after consultation with the FEU, School Examinations and Assessment Council (SEAC), NCVQ and the Training Agency (TA). It proposed six core skills in two groups:

Group 1:   1. Communication; 2. Problem solving; 3. Personal skills;
Group 2:   4. Numeracy; 5. IT; 6. Competence in a modern language.

The first group was to be developed in all post-16 programmes and in every A- and AS-level syllabus. It also recommended the use of Individual Action Plans (IAPs) and the incorporation of National Curriculum themes in the post-16 curriculum with the addition of scientific and technological understanding and aesthetic and creative understanding.

1990: *A British Baccalaureate: Ending the Division Between Education and Training* published by the Institute for Public Policy Research (IPPR). This proposed a unitary 'advanced diploma' delivered through a tertiary college system.

1991: Training and Enterprise Councils (TECs) established. There are 82 TECs. They are limited companies governed by local industrialists and are charged with identifying local training needs and organizing training to meet these needs. They operate government training schemes such as YT. They were announced by the Government in 1988.

1991: White Paper *Education and Training for the 21st Century*. In this review of the education and training system for 16- to 19-year-olds, equal status was demanded for academic and vocational qualifications. Young people 'should not have their opportunities limited by out of date distinctions between qualifications and institutions' (DES 1991: 58). The paper argued that:

> Colleges lack the full freedom which we gave to the polytechnic and higher education colleges in 1989 to respond to the demands of students and the labour market. The Government intend to legislate to remove all colleges of further education . . . and sixth form colleges . . . from local authority control . . . Our policies over the last decade have not done much to enrich that preparation – for life and work.
>
> (DES 1991: 64–5)

1991: National Education and Training Targets (NETTs) set by the government but recommended by the CBI in *World Class Targets* (1991). There was a major review of the targets in 1995.

1992: Further and Higher Education Act. The polytechnics are granted university status. The binary division was subsequently ended when polytechnics became universities in 1993. The CNAA was to be abolished and separate funding councils to be set up for FE and HE.

1992: Education (Schools) Act created the Office for Standards in Education (Ofsted).

1992: GNVQs introduced. Unlike NVQs, these qualifications would be based in schools and colleges rather than the workplace. Level 3 (later 'Advanced') GNVQ was to be 'equivalent' or 'comparable' to A levels. By 1997 students with GNVQs had a greater chance of obtaining a university place than A-level students.

1993: The Department for Education's (DfE) *Charter for Further Education.* This set out rights and expectations and ended with how to complain about 'courses qualifications and results' (pp. 24–9 gives 23 addresses and telephone numbers). All colleges were required to produce their own charters.

1993: incorporation of colleges. The 1992 Further and Higher Education Act was implemented on 1 April. Colleges were taken out of the control of the LEAs and became independent business corporations. Some had turnovers which put them in the *Financial Times* list of big companies. One college had a turnover of almost £50 million.

1994: White Paper *Competitiveness: Helping Business to Win.* Michael Heseltine sets the theme of national competitiveness and calls for improved careers guidance for young people.

1994: Teacher Training Agency (TTA). The Agency was established in September under the directorship of Chief Executive Anthea Millett 'to improve the quality of teaching, to raise the standards of teacher education and training, and to promote teaching as a profession, in order to improve the standards of pupil's achievement and the quality of their learning' (TTA 1995: 7).

1994: new contracts dispute at its height. The FE colleges experienced over three years of action over the introduction of new contracts for lecturers and the abandonment of the so-called 'Silver Book' which set out conditions of service.

1994: Report of the Commission on Social Justice. This report contains the genesis of what would become the 1997 Labour government's views on education and social policy for the 1990s and beyond.

1995: Further Education Development Agency (FEDA) formed. Launched on 7 April, FEDA inherited the staff of the FEU and the Further Education Staff College at Blagdon. Its main function was to 'help FE institutions provide what their student and other customers want and need'. As 'an independent body promoting quality in FE', FEDA intended 'not just to promote best practice but also embody it' (FEDA 1995: 1). Its key aims were to promote quality in teaching and learning, to provide leadership in curriculum design and development, and to ensure effective management.

1995: the Department for Education and Department for Employment merge in July to become the DfEE.

1996: Dearing's *Review of Qualifications for 16–19 Year Olds.* This is Dearing's second much publicized report (Dearing II). Dearing II went for stability and did not recommend a unified system to replace the three existing tertiary qualifications NVQs, GNVQs, and A levels. It did suggest the incorporation of 'key skills' in all three qualifications and the relaunch of YT, modern apprenticeships and the National Record of Achievement. It also suggested that Advanced GNVQs be renamed applied A levels.

Dearing's first report (Dearing I) *The National Curriculum and its Assessment* (1993) was a response to industrial action by teachers throughout the country concerned about the burden of assessment and the narrowness of the National Curriculum. Dearing I reduced time spent on the National Curriculum by 20 per cent and reduced the number of attainment targets and their related statements (SATs). It included a vocational option at Key Stage 4.

1996: the European 'Year of Lifelong Learning'.

1996: *Lifetime Learning* **(DfEE).** A consultation document drawing on previously published work including *Competitiveness: Forging Ahead: Education and Training* (DfEE 1995a). The Labour Party published *Lifelong Learning*, a consultative document (1996).

1996: awarding bodies combine. In 1996, BTEC and London Examinations formed Edexcel. In 1998 C&G, The Associated Examining Board and the Northern Examinations and Assessment Board formed the Assessment and Qualifications Alliance (AQA).

1996: New Labour leader Tony Blair's 'Education, Education and Education' speech to the Labour Party conference on 1 October, 20 years after Callaghan's Ruskin College Speech. The speech was published in *The Times Educational Supplement* of 4 October (p. 6) and some extracts follow.

> Ask me my three main priorities for Government, and I tell you: education, education and education . . . At every level we need radical improvement and reform. A teaching profession trained and able to stand alongside the best in the world and valued as such . . . There should be zero tolerance of failure in Britain's schools. The Age of Achievement will be built on new technology. Our aim is for every school to have access to the superhighway, the computers to deliver it and the education programmes to go on it. With the University for Industry for adult skills, this adds up to a national grid for learning for Britain. Britain the skill superpower of the world.

Task 9.6

Lifelong or lifetime learning, the learning society; why have the phrases become the pre-millennial buzz-words? Can we give them more than rhetorical substance? In what sense is lifelong learning a reality for young people? What features of British society in the 1990s and beyond reveal evidence for the need to become a 'learning society'?

1997: Report of Helena Kennedy's committee of enquiry into widening participation in education *Learning Works.* Kennedy initially suggested redistributing resources and removing the bias towards undergraduates and school sixth forms. Seventy-five per cent of the 5 million students in England are supported by £3.5 billion of funding through the 'Cinderella' service of FE colleges, whereas the university sector with 25 per cent of the student population receives 75 per cent of the available funding. The shocking fact is that 'Sixty-four per cent of university students come from social classes 1 and 2. One per cent come from social class 5' (Kennedy 1997a). The general direction of the many recommendations of the report is a lifetime entitlement to education up to A-level standard, with free teaching for people from deprived backgrounds or with no previous qualifications: 'The government should . . . give priority in public funding within post-16 learning to general education and transferable vocational learning, including key skills, at and leading to level 3: the costs of ensuring that all can succeed to (NVQ) level 3 must be recognised' (Kennedy 1997b: 43).

1997: Publication of the Dearing Report: *Higher Education in the Learning Society, National Committee Inquiry into Higher Education.* One of the nine 'principles' governing the report (Dearing III, Dearing 1997) was that: 'Learning should be increasingly responsive to employment needs and include the development of general skills, widely valued in employment' (Summary Report p. 5). Dearing III was hailed as the most comprehensive review of HE since the Robbins Report. Dearing III made 93 recommendations. These include: a system by which students pay fees covering up to 25 per cent of the cost of tuition (Ch. 20); the establishment of an Institute for Learning and Teaching (ILT) in Higher Education to accredit training programmes for HE staff and to look at computer-based learning (Ch. 8); the promotion of student learning as a high priority (Ch. 8); and a review of research which may allow some institutions to opt out of the competitive funding system based on the Research Assessment Exercise (RAE). In his introduction Dearing sees 'historic boundaries between vocational and academic education breaking down, with increasingly active partnerships between higher education institutions and the worlds of industry commerce and public service' (Summary Report p. 2).

1997: government announces the abolition of student grants and the introduction of fee payments of up to £1000 per annum. The power to do this is given through the Teaching and Higher Education Bill (see below).

1997: NCVQ/School Curriculum and Assessment Authority (SCAA) merge to form a new national curriculum advisory body, the Qualifications and Curriculum Authority (QCA). Its powers are a cause of concern to the awarding bodies.

1997: *Learning for the Twenty-First Century.* In November, Professor Bob Fryer produced the report for the National Advisory Group for Continuing Education and Lifelong Learning. This report consolidates much of the thinking about lifelong learning that has appeared since the Report of the Commission on Social Justice.

1997: Teaching and Higher Education Bill. This bill was the first of a series of responses by the government to Dearing III. It gave the secretary of state powers to interfere in university affairs and is seen by some as a major attack on academic autonomy.

1998: formation of a General Teaching Council (GTC). A GTC was established in Scotland as a result of the Wheatley Report (1963). A voluntary GTC (England and Wales) has been in existence since 1988 and has sought support from the various professional bodies and attempted to secure legislation. The Teaching and Higher Education Bill (1997) established a statutory GTC which will not be a 'teachers' GTC but will have a broad membership. Teachers in schools may now register with the GTC.

1998: *The Learning Age: a renaissance for a new Britain* (DfEE). The expected White Paper on lifelong learning appeared as a Green Paper. It promised to bring learning into the home and workplace.

1998: *Higher Education for the Twenty-First Century: Response to the Dearing Report.* This paper sets out as a priority reaching out to groups underrepresented in higher education. It argues for a better balance between teaching, research and scholarship. An Institute for Learning and Teaching in Higher Education is to be established to accredit programmes of training for HE teachers. Work experience is to become a feature of higher education courses and the aim of employability is stressed.

1998: A University for Industry established after discussions with 'learning organizations' such as Ford, Unipart and Anglian Water. This is not a physical but a virtual university, a network providing access to training.

1999: Hello DOLLY.

> . . . what ought to matter most, in my view, to a learning prime minister is that there should be a powerful Whitehall department responsible for promoting learning across society. This department should be a great office of state on a par with the Foreign Office or the Home Office. If the learning society is to be a reality, nothing else will do. I would want to see the DfEE remain one department, but to change its name – symbolically but importantly – to the Department of Lifelong Learning. It could even be called DOLLY for short. Goodbye DfEE, as it were, Hello . . .
>
> (Barber 1996: 296)

Task 9.7

Having read the chronology, use your general knowledge of history, and the outlines given in the boxed sections, to connect major historical events with particular pieces of legislation and their associated developments in the educational sphere. If you do this, patterns emerge. For example, the three historical periods, 1870–1902, 1902–45, 1945– the present, can be seen as illustrating an almost seamless development in which elementary, then secondary, then further or higher education became a reality for many people. However, also taking 1870 as a starting point we can identify three historical periods: 1870–1914, 1914–39 and 1939– the present, that are sometimes seen as key periods in Britain's relative decline (Sked 1987; Gamble 1990).

Historical periods showing the general developments in PCE can be also be identified. Draw up a chart showing the broad changes in this area over the last 100 years. To do this, identify clearly the different forms of PCE that were provided, the social policy behind that provision and the relevant dates. This will be easier if the tasks of describing the education and training opportunities available to a young person at a given historical moment have been completed. Compare your chart with Table 9.1.

Table 9.1 Developments in PCE

Period	Social policy	Educational provision
Nineteenth century	Little state intervention	Mechanics' institutes
1900–45	Training through 'stop gap' measures	Evening institutes, technical schools
1945–76	Stop gap measures, social orientation, consensus	Day release, technical colleges
1976–90	Crisis, vocationalism, the new vocationalism	FE colleges, training schemes
1990–the present	Crisis and containment	Expansion of FE and HE

Task 9.8

Draw up a brief chronology of key events and reports in your own area of subject or professional expertise. This need not be very detailed. How do key developments correlate with those outlined in the chronology?

Task 9.9

Your chronology is not fixed and should be kept up to date and extended. Further historical details can be added or deleted as your interests, understanding and ideas develop. Add major events and developments as they occur.

9.4 *A comparative chronology: the USA*

Comparative studies of any country might be of academic interest but they usually reflect broader concerns. Traditionally, comparisons were made with Britain's imperial rivals: Germany, the USA and Japan. Between the two World Wars and during the cold war period comparisons with the Soviet education system were common. Here the USA has been chosen but for different reasons. It might be fashionable to look at countries with more dynamic economies and promote aspects of their education. However, the USA is the model for a country attempting to combat its relative economic decline and, at the time of writing, having some success with a 'Goldilocks' economic strategy: not too hot and not too cold, but, like her porridge, 'just right'. That is why government officials and ministers flock to study American policy developments in every sphere. We believe that educational developments in the USA are worthy of study because what happens there usually intimates what will happen in British education at all levels. Therefore it is useful to watch developments that might influence the post-compulsory sector. Indeed some radical thinkers actively promote the American 'community college' system as a model for Britain. Models from other countries are also promoted, in particular the French baccalaureate (BAC) because of its breadth. The French education system has had more extensive and systematic state involvement and direction than the British system traditionally had and is therefore a model for those looking for centralized guidance within a dirigiste philosophy. However informative such a comparison might be in the context of a united Europe, we argue that developments in the USA are more likely to indicate the direction of British educational thinking. Task 9.10 has been designed to test this assumption.

The chronology of vocationally-related acts and events in the history of education in the USA is necessarily very brief. It also covers federal rather than local initiatives and developments in particular states.

9.5 *A chronology of vocational education in the USA*

1862: Land Grant College (Morrill) Act. This provided more public land for the building of colleges. These were now required to train students in military tactics.

1870: Junior Colleges. These two-year 'freshman-sophomore' schools were established before the Civil War but developed rapidly afterwards. The first public junior college was established in 1902.

1896: Dewey's Laboratory School (University Elementary School) established at the University of Chicago. One of Dewey's experiments was with a curriculum centred on the occupations.

1916: Dewey's *Democracy and Education* published. Dewey's book is the most influential work in the history of American education.

1917: Smith-Hughes Act. Aimed at young people aged 14 or over this act brought vocational education into the high school curriculum. It allowed for the training of vocational teachers and created a federal board for vocational education.

1918: schooling becomes compulsory in all states.

1937: George-Deen Act. The federal expenditure on vocational training was more than doubled under this legislation.

1938: Dewey's *Experience and Education* published. A reply to his critics who held that he had brought American education to its knees (Ryan 1995: 277).

1945: George-Barden Act. This act further increased government spending on vocational education and allowed for the training of vocational guidance counsellors.

1954: *Brown* v. *Board of Education of Topeka*. Segregation in American education was outlawed as a result of this case.

1958: National Defense Education Act (NDEA). As a direct result of the launch of 'Sputnik' by the Russians billions of dollars were spent on mathematics, science and modern foreign language education. Funding was to be matched by individual states.

1962: Manpower Training and Development Act. This act was aimed at updating the skills of the hard-core unemployed. Four out of five people who completed the training obtained work.

1963: Vocational Education Act. Federal grants were provided for vocational facilities. Grants went to specialist work-related training schools, high school departments and to schools offering continuing education for full-time workers.

1965: 'Head Start' introduced as a summer programme. It was expanded by 'Follow Through' in 1967.

1969: community/junior colleges cater for over 2 million students.

1971: *Carnegie Commission on Higher Education* calls for the further expansion of two-year community colleges.

1982: Job Training Partnership Act.

1983: Report of the National Commission on Excellence in Education: *A Nation at Risk: The Imperative for Educational Reform.* In contrast to the vocational slant of much of British thinking, this report emphasized the need for academic excellence as a spur to economic recovery. After the 'back to basics' movement of the 1970s it targeted 'new basics' in the form of traditional subjects and 'computer sciences'.

1984: Carl D. Perkins Vocational Education Act. Like the Job Training Partnership Act, this act focused on schemes for the young unemployed.

1990: Commission on the Skills of the American Workforce: *America's Choice: High Skills or Low Wages.*

1990: Carl D. Perkins Vocational and Applied Technology Education Act. This act set out competence-based standards for academic and vocational education.

1991: *America 2000.* This report identified six goals for education: to improve young children's willingness to learn; to increase the numbers graduating from high school; the achievement of grade targets in all subjects; to have students achieve world-class standards in science and mathematics; to ensure every adult is literate and skilled and to free schools and colleges from drugs and violence.

1992: National Educational Goals Panel. This panel reports annually on the achievement of the goals set out in *America 2000.*

Task 9.10

In the American chronology we can detect many parallels with historical developments in Britain. There is an important difference in that there is a recent trend which appears to be a move away from vocationalism to an emphasis on 'new basics' which seem to reflect traditional education values. One writer has gone so far as to say that all the interesting curricular challenges of vocationalism have been lost because 'advocates of vocational education in the USA have so completely capitulated in the face of perceived threats to their existence based on current demands for basics in education' (Lewis 1991: 106). Is this true, or do the demands for the 'new basics' merely reflect the new requirements for workers in the 1990s and beyond to be knowledgeable, self-directing, divergent and adaptable thinkers?

To resolve this and to test whether these developments will filter through to Britain read any articles on current issues in American education in magazines such as *Time* and *Newsweek* and identify any general themes that might be applicable to debates in Britain. There are also some useful Web sites with regularly updated reports and discussions that can be visited, for example: http://www.house.gov/eeo (House Committee on Education and the Workforce); http://ncrve.berkeley.edu (National Center for Research in Vocational Education); http://www.acenet.edu (American Council on Education).

Task 9.11

A small-scale research project: discuss with your fellow students, colleagues and your tutor an issue in PCE that has caught your interest. You will need to identify a fairly narrow area for study. Before you undertake any research always talk the question through with as many people as possible. Ask them and yourself, 'Why is this important?' The more specific the research topic the more informative and useful the research will be. For example, 'Future developments in NVQs' as a topic is too vague and speculative. 'Are the IPPR proposals for a British baccalaureate educationally sound?' is better. Likewise 'The role of government quangos in PCE' is too vast a topic. 'The role and influence of the FEDA on further education' is more manageable.

Task 9.12

It is useful to read texts written in different decades to get a flavour of the time. This runs counter to the fashionable desire to have only the most up to date texts in an academic reading list. The result is a loss of any sense of history. Here is a very limited selection.

For government reports and acts J. Stuart Maclure's *Educational Documents: England and Wales* first published in 1965 is an excellent source. For the period up to 1945 H.C. Barnard's *A History of English Education* (1947) and W.H.G. Armytage's *Four Hundred Years of English Education* (Cambridge University Press, 1964) are full of detail. They need some supplementing, as they are general histories of education (cf. Coffey 1992; Skilbeck *et al.* 1994: 156–62).

Chapters 1 and 8 of W.O. Lester Smith's *Education* (Penguin, 1957) provide some clear thinking and an interesting comparison with today's debates on education, industry and citizenship.

For an understanding of how the new vocationalism was contested Dan Finn's *Training Without Jobs* (Macmillan, 1987) is good, as is Cynthia Cockburn's *Twin Track Training* (Macmillan, 1987) which looks at sex inequalities in YTS.

Pat Ainley's work, such as *Vocational Education and Training* (Cassell, 1990), is an attempt to describe a form of vocational education which meets what he perceives as the needs of the working class.

Analysis of developments as a result of the incorporation of the FE colleges in 1993 is difficult because the best sources are ephemeral magazines and bulletins. One source is the journal *General Educator* (edited by Colin Waugh for the NATFHE General Education Section). Each edition contains a summary of literature and events and discussions of the conflicts and disputes that are written out of most books.

A sound critique of competence-based training is Terry Hyland's *Competence Education and NVQs: Dissenting Perspectives* (Cassell, 1994).

A good book to start you thinking about issues in the 1990s such as postmodernism and globalization as they are believed to affect PCE is James Avis and his colleagues' *Knowledge and Nationhood: Education, Politics and Work* (Cassell, 1996).

BIBLIOGRAPHY

Ahier, J. and Ross, A. (1995) *The Social Subjects Within the Curriculum.* London: Falmer Press.

Ainley, P. (1988) *From School to YTS: Education and Training in England and Wales 1944–1987.* Milton Keynes: Open University Press.

Ainley, P. (1990) *Vocational Education and Training.* London: Cassell.

Ainley, P. (1993) *Class and Skill: Changing Divisions of Knowledge and Labour.* London: Cassell.

Ainley, P. (1994) *Degrees of Difference: Higher Education in the 1990s.* London: Lawrence & Wishart.

Ainscow, M. and Tweddle, D. (1988) *Preventing Classroom Failure.* London: David Fulton Publishers Ltd.

Anderson, J. (1980a) Socrates as educator, in D.Z. Phillips (ed.) *Education and Inquiry*, pp. 64–80. London: Basil Blackwell.

Anderson, J. (1980b) Lectures on the educational theories of Spencer and Dewey, in D.Z. Phillips (ed.) *Education and Inquiry*, pp. 81–141. London: Basil Blackwell.

Anderson, J. (1980c) Education and practicality, in D.Z. Phillips (ed.) *Education and Inquiry*, pp. 153–8. London: Basil Blackwell.

Annan, N. (1990) *Our Age: The Generation That Made Post-war Britain.* London: Fontana.

Aristotle (1904) *The Politics*, Book VIII, trans. T.A. Sinclair. Harmondsworth: Penguin.

Armytage, W.H.G. (1970) *Four Hundred Years of English Education.* Cambridge: Cambridge University Press.

Association of University Teachers (1997) AUT Bulletin, April.

Avis, J., Bloomer, M., Esland, G., Gleeson, D. and Hodkinson, P. (1996) *Knowledge and Nationhood: Education, Politics and Work.* London: Cassell.

Ball, S. (1987) *The Micro-Politics of the School.* London: Methuen.

Barber, M. (1996) *The Learning Game.* London: Victor Gollancz.

Barnes, D. (1982) *Practical Curriculum Study.* London: Routledge and Kegan Paul.

Barrow, R. (1984) *Giving teaching back to teachers: a critical introduction to curriculum theory.* Brighton: Wheatsheaf.

Beaumont, G. (1995) *Review of 100 NVQs and SVQs*. London: DfEE.

Bell, J. (1987) *Doing Your Research Project*. Milton Keynes: Open University Press.

Benn, C. and Chitty, C. (1997) *Thirty Years On: Is Comprehensive Education Alive and Well or Struggling to Survive?* Harmondsworth: Penguin.

Benn, C. and Fairley, J. (eds) (1986) *Challenging the MSC on Jobs, Training and Education*. London: Pluto Press.

Bennett, N. and McNamara, D. (1979) *Focus on Teaching*. London: Longman.

Bloom, A. (1991) Introduction, in *Rousseau's Emile or On Education*. Harmondsworth: Penguin.

Bloom, B.S. (1964) *Taxonomy of Educational Objectives: Handbook 1/Cognitive Domain*. London: Longman.

Boden, M.A. (1994) *Piaget*. London: Fontana.

Boyd, W. (1956) *Emile for Today: The Emile of Jean-Jacques Rousseau*, selected, translated and interpreted by William Boyd. London: Heinemann.

Brookfield, S. (1986) *Understanding and Facilitating Learning*. Milton Keynes: Open University Press.

Brooks, R. (1991) *Contemporary Debates in Education: An Historical Perspective*. London: Longman.

Buchanan, S. (ed.) (1982) Introduction, in *The Portable Plato*. Harmondsworth: Penguin.

Calderhead, J. (1987) *Exploring Teachers' Thinking*. London: Cassell.

Capey, J. (1995) *GNVQ Assessment Review: Final Report of the Review Group*. London: NCVQ.

Chickering, A.W. and Havighurst, R. (1981) The life cycle, in A.W. Chickering (ed.) *The Modern American College*. San Francisco, CA: Jossey-Bass.

Child, D. (1993) *Psychology and the Teacher*. London: Cassell.

Cockburn, C. (1987) *Two Track Training: Sex Inequalities and the YTS*. London: Macmillan.

Coffey, D. (1992) *Schools and Work*. London: Cassell.

Coffield, F. (1997) Prophets of the true god, *Times Educational Supplement*, 24 January.

Cohen, L. and Manion, L. (1989) *Research Methods in Education*. London: Routledge.

Corbett, J. and Barton, L. (1992) *A Struggle for Choice*. London: Routledge.

Cornwall, J. (1996) *Choice, Opportunity and Learning*. London: Fulton.

Corson, D. (ed.) (1991) *Education for Work*. Clevedon, Avon: Multilingual Matters Ltd.

Coulby, D. and Jones, C. (1995) *Postmodernity and European Education Systems*. Stoke-on-Trent: Trentham Books.

Cronbach, L.J. (1980) *Toward Reform of Program Evaluation*. San Francisco: Jossey-Bass.

CSJ (Commission on Social Justice) (1994) *Social Justice: Strategies for National Renewal*. London: Vintage.

Curzon, L.B. (ed.) (1990) *Teaching in Further Education*, 4th edn. London: Cassell.

Daunt, P. (1991) *Meeting Disability: A European Response*. London: Cassell.

Davies, W.J.K. (1975) *Learning Resources*. London: Council for Educational Technology.

Dearing, R. (1996) *Review of Qualifications for 16–19 Year Olds* (Dearing II). Hayes: SCAA.

Dearing, R. (1997) *Higher Education in the Learning Society: Report of the National Committee of Inquiry into Higher Education* (Dearing III). London: HMSO.

DES (1991) *Education and Training for the 21st Century*, Cmnd. 1536. London: HMSO.

Dewey, J. (1915) *The School and Society*. Chicago: University of Chicago Press.

Dewey, J. ([1916] 1966) *Democracy and Education*. New York: Macmillan/The Free Press.

Dewey, J. ([1938] 1971) *Experience and Education*. New York: Collier Books.

DfEE (1995a) *Competitiveness: Forging Ahead Education and Training*. London: HMSO.

DfEE (1995b) *Lifetime Learning: A Consultation Document*. London: HMSO.

DfEE (1998) *Higher Education for the 21st Century: Response to the Dearing Report*. London: DfEE.

Dickinson, L. (1992) *Learner Autonomy*. Dublin: Authentik.

Donald, J. (1992) *Sentimental Education*. London: Verso.

Dunnill, R., Nakarada, S. and Raffo, C. (1995) An Approach to the Revised Advanced Business GNVQ. *Economics and Business Education*, 3 (11): 135.

Egan, G. (1994) *The Skilled Helper*. Pacific Grove, CA: Brooks/Cole Publishing Co.

Ellington, H. and Race, P. (1993) *Producing Teaching Materials*, 2nd edn. London: Kogan Page.

Ellington, H., Percival, F. and Race, P. (1993) *Handbook of Educational Technology* 3rd edn. London: Kogan Page.

Elliott, J. (1993) Introduction in J. Elliott (ed.) *Reconstructing Teacher Education*. London: Falmer Press.

Engels, F. ([1878] 1975) *Anti-Duhring*. London: Lawrence and Wishart.

Farish, M., McPake, J., Powney, J. and Weiner, G. (1996) *Equal Opportunities in Colleges and Universities*. Buckingham: The Society for Research into Higher Education & Open University Press.

FEDA (1995) *Launch Newsletter*, May. London: FEDA.

FEFC (1996) *Quality and Standards in Further Education in England: Chief Inspector's Annual Report 1995–96*. Coventry: FEFC.

FEU (Further Education Unit) (1987) *Marketing Adult and Continuing Education: A Project Report*. London: FEU.

Finegold, D.N. and Soskice, D. (1988) The failure of training in Britain: analysis and prescription. *Oxford Review of Economic Policy*, 4 (3): 21–53.

Finegold, D.N., Keep, E., Milliband, D., Raffe, D., Spours, K. and Young, M. (1990) *A British Baccalaureate*. London: IPPR.

Finn, D. (1986) YTS: the jewel in the MSC's crown? in C. Benn and J. Fairley (eds) *Challenging the MSC on Jobs, Training and Education*. London: Pluto Press.

Finn, D. (1987) *Training without Jobs: New Deals and Broken Promises*. London: Macmillan.

Francis, D. and Young, D. (1979) *Improving Working Groups*. London: University Association.

Fryer, R.H. (1997) *Learning for the 21st Century: First Report of the National Advisory Group for Continuing Education and Lifelong Learning*. London: NAGCELL.

Gagné, R. (1977) *Conditions of Learning*. New York: Holt, Rinehart and Winston.

Gamble, A. (1990) *Britain in Decline: Economic Policy, Political Strategy and the British State*, 3rd edn. London: Macmillan.

Gibbs, G., Habeshaw, S. and Habeshaw, T. (1988) *53 Interesting Ways to Appraise Your Teaching*. Bristol: Technical and Educational Services Ltd.

Gibbs, G. and Habeshaw, T. (1989) *Preparing to Teach*. Bristol: Technical and Educational Services Ltd.

Gibbs, G. and Parsons, C. (1994) *Course Design for Resource Based Learning*. Oxford: Oxford Centre for Staff Development.

Gilroy, P. (1993) Reflections on Schon, in P. Gilroy and M. Smith (eds) *International Analyses of Teacher Education*. Abingdon: Carfax, Journal of Education and Training Papers 1.

Glennerster, N. (1995) *British Social Policy Since 1945*. London: Basil Blackwell.

Goodson, I.F. (1994) *Studying Curriculum: Cases and Methods*. Buckingham: Open University Press.

Goodson, I.F. and Hargreaves, A. (eds) (1996) *Teachers' Professional Lives*. London: Falmer Press.

Hall, V. (1994) *Further Education in the UK*, 2nd edn. London and Bristol: Collins Educational and The Staff College.

Hamilton, D. (1976) *Curriculum Evaluation*. London: Open Books.

Hargreaves, A. (1994) *Changing Teachers, Changing Times: Teachers' Work and Culture in a Postmodern Age*. London: Cassell.

Hearnshaw, L.S. (1979) *Cyril Burt, Psychologist*. London: Hodder & Stoughton.

Hickox, M. (1995) Situating vocationalism. *British Journal of Sociology of Education*, 16 (2): 153–62.

Higham, J., Sharp, P. and Yeomans, D. (1996) *The Emerging 16–19 Curriculum*. London: Fulton.

Hirst, P.H. ([1965] 1973) Liberal education and the nature of knowledge, in R.S. Peters (ed.) *The Philosophy of Education*. Oxford: Oxford University Press.

Hirst, P.H. (1974) *Knowledge and the Curriculum*. London: Routledge and Kegan Paul.

Hirst, P.H. (1993) Education, knowledge and practices, in R. Barrow and P. White (eds) *Beyond Liberal Education: Essays in Honour of Paul H. Hirst*, pp. 184–99. London: Routledge.

HMSO (1959) *15–18: A Report of the Central Advisory Council for Education/England* (Crowther Report). London: HMSO.

HMSO (1986) *The National Council for Vocational Qualifications: Its Purposes and Aims*. London: HMSO.

Hoggart, R. (1996) *The Way We Live Now*. London: Pimlico.

Holland, R.F. (1980) *Against Empiricism: On Education, Epistemology and Value*, pp. 2–25. London: Basil Blackwell.

Hopkins, D. (1989) *Evaluation for School Development*. Milton Keynes: Open University Press.

Houle, C.O. (1961) *The Enquiring Mind*. Madison: University of Wisconsin Press.

Houle, C.O. (1972) *The Design of Education*. San Francisco: Jossey-Bass.

Huddleston, P. and Unwin, L. (1997) *Teaching and Learning in Further Education: Diversity and Change*. London: Routledge.

Hudson, A., Hayes, D. and Andrew, T. (1996) *Working Lives in the 1990s*. London: Global Futures.

Hudson, L. (1966) *Contrary Imaginations*. London: Methuen.

Hyland, T. (1994) *Competence, Education and NVQs: Dissenting Perspectives*. London: Cassell.

IRDAC (1990) *Skills Shortages in Europe*. Industrial Research and Advisory Committee.

Jackson, P.W. (1968) *Life in Classrooms*. New York: Hall, Rinehart & Winston.

Jarvis, P. (1995) *Adult and Continuing Education Theory and Practice*. London: Routledge.

Kennedy, H. (1997a) *Guardian*, 27 May, 1997.

Kennedy, H. (1997b) *Learning Works: Widening Participation in Further Education*. Coventry: FEFC.

Knowles, M. (1984) *The Adult Learner, a Neglected Species*, 3rd edn. Houston, TX: Gulf Publishing Company.

Kolb, D. (1984) *Experiential Learning: Experience as a Source of Learning and Development*. New York: Prentice Hall.

Korndörffer, W. (1991) Vocational skills training in transition education, in D. Corson (ed.) *Education for Work*, pp. 220–31. Clevedon, Avon: Multilingual Matters Ltd.

Krol, E. (1994) *The Whole Internet*. Sebastopal, CA: O'Reilly & Associates.

Labour Party (1996) *Road to the Manifesto: Lifelong Learning*. London: The Labour Party.

Langenbach, M. (1988) *Curriculum Models in Adult Education*. Malabar, FL: Krieger Publishing.

Lawton, D. (1983) *Curriculum Studies and Educational Planning*. London: Hodder and Stoughton.

Leicester, M. (1994) Competence, knowledge and education: reply to Hyland. *Journal of Philosophy of Education*, 28 (1): 113–18.

Lewis, T. (1991) Difficulties attending the new vocationalism in the USA. *Journal of the Philosophy of Education*, 25 (1): 95–108.

Lewis, T. (1997) Towards a liberal education. *Journal of the Philosophy of Education*, 3 (3): 477–90.

Locke, J. ([1693] 1989) *Some Thoughts Concerning Education*. Oxford: Clarendon Press.

Lovell, R.B. (1980) *Adult Learning*. London: Croom Helm.

Maclure, J.S. (1965) *Educational Documents: England and Wales*. London: Chapman and Hall, reprinted by Methuen, London and New York.

Maclure, S. (1988) *Education Reformed: A Guide to the Education Reform Act*. London: Hodder and Stoughton.

McGivney, V. (1990) *Access to Education for Non-Participating Adults*. Leicester: NIACE.

McIntyre, D., Hagger, H. and Wilkin, M. (eds) *Mentoring: Perspectives on School-Based Teacher Education*. London: Kogan Page.

McNamara, B. (1979) *Focus on Teaching*. London: Longman.

Marx, K. ([1867] 1974) *Capital*, vol. 1. London: Lawrence & Wishart.

Marx, K. ([1875] 1968) Critique of the Gotha Programme, in K. Marx and F. Engels, *Selected Works*. London: Lawrence & Wishart.

Maslow, A.H. (1970) *Motivation and Personality*. New York: Harper and Row.

Maynard, T. and Furlong, J. (1993) Learning to teach and models of mentoring, in D. McIntyre, H. Hagger and M. Wilkin (eds) *Mentoring: Perspectives on School-based Teacher Education*. London: Kogan Page.

Minton, D. (1991) *Teaching Skills in Further and Adult Education*. Basingstoke: City & Guilds/Macmillan.

Moore, M. (1983) On a theory of independent study, in D. Sewart, D. Keegan and B. Holmberg (eds) *Distance Education: International Perspectives*, pp. 68–94. London: Croom Helm.

Napier, R.W. and Gershenfeld, M.K. (1989) *Groups, Theory and Experience*. 4th edn. Boston: Houghton Mifflin.

National Commission on Education (1993) *Learning to Succeed: Report of the Peter Hamlyn Foundation*. London: Heinemann.

NCVQ (1988) *Information Leaflet Number 1*. London: NCVQ.

Nuttall, L. (1988) Transmitted, caught or taught? A whole school approach to personal and social education. *Pastoral Care*, March.

Passmore, J. (1973) On teaching to be critical, in R.S. Peters (ed.) *The Concept of Education*, pp. 192–211. London: Routledge and Kegan Paul.

Perkinson, H.J. (1980) *Since Socrates: Studies in the History of Western Educational Thought*. London: Longman.

Phillips, M. (1996) *All Must Have Prizes*. London: Little, Brown and Company.

Pincas, A. (1997) IT Focus, *Guardian*, 27 May.

Plato [1993] *The Apology*, in H. Tarrant (ed.) *The Last Days of Socrates*. Harmondsworth: Penguin.

Plato [1956] *Protagoras and Meno*. Translated by W.K.C. Guthrie. Harmondsworth: Penguin.

Plato, *Republic*. In *The Portable Plato*, edited with an introduction by Scott Buchanan. Harmondsworth: Penguin, 1982.

Powell, R. (1991) *Resources for Flexible Learning*. Stafford: Network Education Press.

Preedy, M. (1989) *Approaches to Curriculum Management*. Milton Keynes: Open University Press.

Pring, R. (1992) Liberal education and vocational preparation, in William (eds) *Continuing the Education Debate*, pp. 54–64. London: Cassell.

Pring, R. (1993) Liberal education and vocational preparation, in R. Barrow and P. White (eds) *Beyond Liberal Education: Essays in Honour of Paul H. Hirst*, pp. 49–78. London: Routledge.

Race, P. (1992) *53 Interesting Ways to Write Open Learning Materials*. Bristol: Technical and Educational Services Ltd.

Raggatt, P., Edwards, R. and Small, N. (eds) (1966) *The Learning Society, Challenges and Trends*. London: Routledge in association with the Open University.

Reece, I. and Walker, S. (1994) *A Practical Guide to Teaching, Training and Learning*. Sunderland: Business Education Publishing.

Riley, P. (1985) *Discourse and Learning*. London: Longman.

Robbins, Lord L.C. (1963) *Higher Education: Report of the Committee on Higher Education*, Cmnd 2154. London: HMSO.

Roberts, K., Blunden, G. and Ruseborough, G. (1994) Review symposium: class and skill. *British Journal of Sociology of Education*, 15 (1): 119–27.

Robertson, J. (1989) *Effective Classroom Control*. London: Hodder & Stoughton.

Rogers, A. (1996) *Teaching Adults*. Buckingham: Open University Press.

Rogers, C. (1983) *Freedom to Learn for the '80s*. Columbus, Ohio: Merrill.

Rousseau, J.J. ([1762] 1991) *Émile*. Harmondsworth: Penguin.

Rowntree, D. (1987) *Assessing Students: How Shall We Know Them?* London: Kogan Page.

Russell, B. ([1959] 1989) *Wisdom of the West*. London: Bloomsbury.

Ryan, A. (1995) *John Dewey and the High Tide of American Liberalism*. New York: W.W. Norton.

Ryle, G. (1973) Teaching and training, in R.S. Peters (ed.) *The Concept of Education*, pp. 105–19. London: Routledge and Kegan Paul.

Satterly, D. (1990) *Assessment in Schools*. London: Basil Blackwell.

Scrimshaw, P. (1983) *Purpose and Planning in the Classroom*. Milton Keynes: Open University Press.

Simon, B. (1985) Marx and the crisis in education, in *Does Education Matter?*, pp. 173–96. London: Lawrence & Wishart.

Sked, A. (1987) *Britain's Decline: Problems and Perspectives*. London: Basil Blackwell.

Skilbeck, M. (1976) *Curriculum Design and Development*. Milton Keynes: Open University Press.

Skilbeck, M., Connell, H., Lowe, N. and Tait, K. (1994) *The Vocational Quest: New Directions in Education and Training*. London: Routledge.

Skinner, B.F. (1938) *The Behaviour of Organisms: An Experimental Analysis*. New York: Appleton-Century-Crofts.

Skuse, P. (1997) Evidence from Turner's Syndrome of an imprinted X-linked locus affecting cognitive functioning. *Nature*, 387: 705–8.

Smith, W.O. Lester (1957) *Education*. Harmondsworth: Penguin.

Stenhouse, L. (1975) *An Introduction to Curriculum Research and Development*. London: Heinemann.

Sutcliffe, J. (1990) *Adults with Learning Difficulties*. Leicester: NIACE.

Taba, H. (1962) *Curriculum Development: Theory and Practice*. New York: Harcourt Brace.

Tanner, D. and Tanner, L.M. (1980) *Curriculum Development: Theory Into Practice.* New York: Macmillan.

Tarrant, H. (ed.) (1993) *The Last Days of Socrates.* Harmondsworth: Penguin.

Tawney, R.H. (1922) *Secondary Education for All.* Reprinted 1988, London: The Hambledon Press.

Taylor, P.H. and Richards, C.M. (1985) *An Introduction to Curriculum Studies.* Windsor: NFER/Nelson.

Teacher Training Agency (1995) *Corporate Plan 1995: Promoting High Quality Teaching and Teacher Education.* London: TTA.

Tennant, M. (1988) *Psychology and Adult Learning.* London: Routledge.

The Economist (1996) Training and jobs: what works?, 6 April.

Thorndike, E.L. (1912) *Education: A First Book.* New York: Macmillan.

Tight, M. (1996) *Key Concepts in Adult Education and Training.* London: Routledge.

Tight, M. (ed.) (1983) *Adult Learning and Education.* London: Routledge.

Timmins, N. (1996) *The Five Giants: A Biography of the Welfare State.* London: Fontana.

Tough, A. (1979) *The Adult's Learning Projects: A Fresh Approach to Theory and Practice in Adult Learning.* Toronto: Ontario Institute for Studies in Education.

Tyler, R. (1971) *Basic Principles for Curriculum and Instruction.* Chicago: University of Chicago Press.

Walker, D.F. and Soltis, J.F. (1992) *Curriculum and Aims.* London: Teachers College Press.

Walklin, L. (1990) *Teaching and Learning in Further Education.* Cheltenham: Stanley Thornes.

Williams, K. (1994) Vocationalism and liberal education: exploring the tensions. *Journal of Philosophy of Education,* 28 (1): 89–100.

Williams, M. (1992) Ruskin in context, in M. Williams, R. Daugherty and F. Burns (eds) *Continuing the Education Debate.* London: Cassell.

Williams, M., Daugherty, R. and Burns, F. (eds) (1992) *Continuing the Education Debate.* London: Cassell.

Willis, P. (1987) Foreword, in D. Finn (ed.) *Training Without Jobs: New Deals and Broken Promises.* London: Macmillan.

Wolf, A. (1993) *Assessment Issues and Problems in a Criterion-based System.* London: FEU.

Wolf, A. and Black, H. (1990) *Knowledge and Competence: Current Issues in Training and Education.* Sheffield: Careers and Occupational Information Centre.

Woudhuysen, J. (1997) Before we rush to declare a new era, in G. Mulgan (ed.) *Life After Politics,* pp. 352–9. London: Fontana.

Wragg, E.C. (1994) *An Introduction to Classroom Observation.* London: Routledge.

Yaffe, D. (1976) *The State and the Capitalist Crisis.* London: Mimeo.

Youngman, M.B. (1986) *Analysing Questionnaires.* Nottingham: University of Nottingham School of Education, Trentham Books.

INDEX